PRACTICAL ASPECTS
OF SIGNAL DETECTION
IN PHARMACOVIGILANCE

Report of CIOMS Working Group VIII

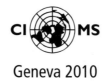

Geneva 2010

ISBN 92 9036 082 8

Acknowledgements

The Council for International Organizations of Medical Sciences (CIOMS) gratefully acknowledges the contributions of the members of the CIOMS Working Group VIII on Practical Aspects of Signal Detection in Pharmacovigilance. Moreover, CIOMS recognizes the generous support of the drug regulatory authorities, pharmaceutical companies and other organizations and institutions which provided their expertise and the resources that resulted in this publication. Each member participated actively in the discussions, drafting and redrafting of texts and their review, which enabled the Working Group to bring the entire project to a successful conclusion.

CIOMS thanks especially those members who chaired the meetings of the Working Group VIII for their dedication and capable leadership. Each of the meetings had a nominated rapporteur and CIOMS acknowledges their professional contributions.

The editorial group, comprising Drs June Raine, Philippe Close, Gerald Dal Pan, Ralph Edwards, Bill Gregory, Manfred Hauben, Atsuko Shibata, June Almenoff, Lynn Macdonald and Stephen Klincewicz, merits special mention and thanks. CIOMS wishes to express special appreciation to Dr June Raine as Chief Editor of the final report.

The contribution by the CIOMS/WHO Working Group on Vaccine Pharmacovigilance of the Points to Consider in Appendix 5 is gratefully acknowledged.

CIOMS and the Working Group are grateful for important input received on several points of the report from senior experts outside the Group who made valuable suggestions: Professor Stephen Evans, Dr Toshiharu Fujita, Dr David Madigan, Dr Niklas Norén, Dr Hironori Sakai, Professor Saad Shakir, Dr Hugh Tilson and Dr Patrick Waller.

Geneva, December 2009

Gottfried Kreutz,
Dr. med., Dipl.-Chem.
Secretary-General, CIOMS

Juhana E. Idänpään-Heikkilä,
MD, PhD, Professor
Senior Adviser, CIOMS

Table of Contents

Preface

In recent years public expectations for rapid identification and prompt management of emerging drug safety issues have grown swiftly. Over a similar timeframe, the move from paper-based adverse event reporting systems to electronic capture and rapid transmission of data has resulted in the accrual of substantial datasets capable of complex analysis and querying by industry, regulators and other public health organizations.

These two drivers have created a fertile environment for pharmacovigilance scientists, information technologists and statistical experts, working together, to deliver novel approaches to detect signals from these extensive and quickly growing datasets, and to manage them appropriately. In following this exciting story, this report looks at the practical consequences of these developments for pharmacovigilance practitioners.

The report aims primarily to provide a comprehensive resource for those considering how to strengthen their pharmacovigilance systems and practices, and to give practical advice. But the report does not specify instant solutions. These will inevitably be situation specific and require careful consideration taking into account local needs. However, the CIOMS Working Group VIII is convinced that the combination of methods and a clear policy on the management of signals will strengthen current systems.

Finally, in looking ahead, the report anticipates a number of ongoing developments, including techniques with wider applicability to other data forms than individual case reports. The ultimate test for pharmacovigilance systems is the demonstration of public health benefit and it is this test which signal detection methodologies need to meet if the expectations of all stakeholders are to be fulfilled.

I

Introduction and scope of CIOMS VIII

A signal in pharmacovigilance was defined by WHO in 2002 as "Reported information on a possible causal relationship between an adverse event and a drug, the relationship being previously unknown or incompletely documented. Usually more than a single case report is required to generate a signal, depending on the seriousness of the event and quality of the information" (*1*). This definition has served the pharmacovigilance community well, as most information about adverse events was obtained via individual case reports submitted from practitioners and patients at the point of care. In recent years, however, information about the safety of medicines has come from a variety of sources, including not only databases of spontaneous individual case reports, but also from electronic medical records, administrative healthcare databases, and clinical trials. Because of these trends, the nature of signal detection, and the very nature of a signal itself, has changed. The CIOMS VIII project was undertaken to address the evolving nature of signal detection in pharmacovigilance.

The objective of the CIOMS VIII report is to provide useful points for consideration to manufacturers, regulatory authorities, international monitoring centers and others wishing to establish or understand the output of a systematic and holistic strategy to better manage the entire "lifecycle" of a drug safety signal. This lifecycle includes signal detection, signal prioritization, and signal evaluation. If the evaluation of a drug safety signal establishes a new adverse drug reaction, then this stage of the signal's lifecycle will lead to an update of the product's prescribing information and, possibly, other regulatory actions including further risk communications and risk minimization efforts.

The concept of a drug safety signal is not new. Indeed, it has been the cornerstone of pharmacovigilance activities for about forty years. However, as more medicines are authorized for marketing each year, and as increasing numbers of persons are taking medicines, this has resulted in an increase in the number of adverse events reported to manufacturers and to regulators. The manual review of paper-based reports that provided the foundation of early productive pharmacovigilance systems is simply no longer practical. Modern pharmacovigilance systems, which receive several hundred thousand reports each year and which have databases containing several million adverse event reports, must be able to detect, prioritize, and evaluate signals in an efficient and proactive manner. To do so requires a systematic approach that couples statistical and analytic methods with sound clinical judgment.

To date in the field of pharmacovigilance, this systematic approach has been applied most widely to post-approval signal detection, prioritization and evaluation using passive surveillance systems collecting spontaneous case reports of suspected adverse drug reactions. Thus, the scope of the CIOMS Working Group VIII concentrates on providing practical, focused, and timely information about the application of these proactive approaches to passive surveillance systems of spontaneous case reports. While this report is not intended to provide an equal amount of attention to signal detection, prioritization and evaluation using active surveillance methods applied to other non-spontaneous sources of post-approval data (including large linked databases of claims data, electronic medical records databases, patient registry data, prescription-event monitoring studies, case-control surveillance studies, and cumulative post-approval meta-analyses of randomized clinical trial data), new developments in this area are summarized. Though application of a systematic approach to signal detection in these databases is less well developed, it is anticipated that their use will become increasingly important in the years to come. Toward that end, we address this topic to provide the reader with a framework for understanding the developments that are expected to come in the next several years.

While randomized clinical trial data are generally thought to accrue from the pre-approval period, there is often a substantial body of randomized clinical trial safety data that accumulates after approval. The data from both pre- and post-approval randomized clinical trials can be pooled in a cumulative meta-analysis to elucidate previously unrecognized adverse drug reactions that the pre-approval human safety database was unable to detect because of insufficient sample size (lack of statistical power) (2, 3). Readers interested in this specific topic should consult the CIOMS Working Group VI report that provides useful recommendations for the management of safety information from clinical trials (4).

It is important to understand the context in which this project was undertaken. First, the development of statistical and analytical techniques to examine databases of adverse event reports does not replace the need for the careful and sound clinical judgment required to detect signals and to assess the possible causal relationship between a drug and an adverse event. These statistical and analytical methods are designed to facilitate signal detection, not provide evidence of causality. Second, the increasing availability of large healthcare databases will not, at least for the foreseeable future, replace the need for spontaneous reporting systems. The accurate recording of careful clinical observations made at the point of care – an essential element of a robust spontaneous surveillance system   cannot be replaced by automated databases. Third, application of a systematic approach to signal detection is an evolving field. New techniques are being developed, and these techniques are being applied to new databases. While there is much enthusiasm about the potential utility of these new approaches and data sources, their value will have to be established.

The audience for this report is broad. It is intended for all those who work in the field of pharmacovigilance. It is not simply limited to pharmacovigilance organizations that have modern passive surveillance systems that collect spontaneous case reports using structured forms (e.g. CIOMS I) and enter these data into large relational databases with uniform data elements (e.g. ICH E2B format) and controlled vocabularies (e.g. MedDRA) that can be queried to generate cross-tabulations of frequency counts of case reports or instances of drug-event combinations in the entire database stratified by key variables (e.g. suspect medication name, MedDRA preferred term, age group, sex, year of report, etc). Rather, the CIOMS Working Group VIII recognizes that many persons and organizations active in pharmacovigilance might not have their own databases, computing capability or statisticians. This report will be of use to those who wish to apply these techniques to publicly available databases, those who are contemplating implementing these techniques in their own databases, and those who will be reviewing the output of such efforts. With this audience in mind, the CIOMS Working Group VIII sought to give as much practical advice as possible. This report is also intended for pharmacoepidemiologists who deal primarily with case-control or cohort studies, but who use data from spontaneous reports, so that they can understand the role and value of the techniques presented in this report in the overall approach to the study of post-marketing drug safety.

Signal detection, prioritization and evaluation are just a few steps in the post-marketing drug safety evaluation schema. Monitoring the effects of public health interventions aimed at minimizing the incidence or severity of the identified adverse drug reaction in the treated patient population is also part of the lifecycle of a drug safety signal as specified in the guidance on risk management systems (5). A comprehensive discussion of risk communication, risk minimization, and regulatory actions resulting from signal detection activities is beyond the scope of this report. However, the timing of such public health interventions along the signal lifecycle is discussed.

The CIOMS VIII report focuses on the lifecycle of drug safety signals for drugs and therapeutic biologicals. The CIOMS/WHO Working Group on Vaccine Pharmacovigilance focuses on terminology and definitions relevant to vaccines. Safety signals related to other types of medical products (e.g. medical devices, blood products, and dietary/herbal supplements) are not covered in this report. The generation and evaluation of safety data for these products is sufficiently different from those of drug and therapeutic biological products that they have been excluded.

References

1. *Safety of medicines: a guide to detecting and reporting adverse drug reactions.* Geneva, WHO, 2002 (http://whqlibdoc.who.int/hq/2002/WHO_EDM_QSM_2002.2.pdf).

2. Nissen SE, Wolski K. Effect of rosiglitazone on risk of myocardial infarction and death from cardiovascular causes. *New England Journal of Medicine*, 2007, 356:2457-71.

3. Singh S, Loke YK, Furberg CD. Long-term risk of cardiovascular events with rosiglitazone: a meta-analysis. *Journal of the American Medical Association*, 2007, 298:1189-95.

4. *Management of Safety Information from Clinical Trials.* Report of CIOMS Working Group VI. Geneva, CIOMS, 2005.

5. *Pharmacovigilance planning,* ICH E2E Guideline, 2004; *Guideline on risk management systems for medicinal products for human use.* EMEA, 2005; and *Development and use of risk minimization action plans,* FDA Guidance, 2005.

II

Background – pharmacovigilance and key definitions

a. Need for pharmacovigilance after regulatory approval

The clinical development process for all new medicines represents a societal and regulatory compromise between two conflicting goals: a) the desire to have adequate evidence requirements that allow patients to have timely access to new efficacious medicines and allow companies to have a period of patent protection to justify their significant research and development investments; and b) the desire to learn as much as possible about a medicine's efficacy and safety prior to approval. As a result, pre-approval clinical trials are not of sufficient size to elucidate and characterize every adverse effect of a medicinal product, and their results cannot be assumed to be generalizable to patients who will use the product in a usual care setting (*1*). CIOMS Working Group VI (*2*) listed the main limitations of a typical pre-approval human safety database as: a) the small numbers of study subjects relative to the much larger and diverse population that may use the product, such that it is not possible to detect rare adverse reactions; b) the statistical aspects of study designs that focus on efficacy endpoint(s) rather than on safety; c) a highly-controlled, experimental environment that may not reflect medical practice in a "real world" setting (protocol-mandated laboratory tests and scheduled visits); d) uncertain generalizability of the results to patients not included in the pre-approval trials (due to concomitant medications, concurrent comorbidities, etc.); and e) a relatively short duration of treatment that would preclude the observation of adverse events with a long latency period (e.g. cancer).

The pre-approval testing of a new drug is generally designed to test the efficacy of the product, as well as to characterize the most common adverse effects of the drug. Most new drugs are approved after a few thousand patients are exposed to them. In some cases, the number studied in pre-approval trials may be much smaller, and in other cases it may be much larger. Once the product is marketed, it generally gets used by a large number of people, often more clinically diverse than those who participated in the pre-approval studies. It is well known that patients studied in clinical trials are generally more highly selected for treatment than are patients who receive the drug once it is marketed. Compared to patients in clinical trials, patients who receive the drug once it is marketed may have more comorbid conditions (including medically serious conditions), may be taking more concomitant medications, may have a wider spectrum of disease severity, or may be using the product for unstudied (off-label) uses.

b. Definition of pharmacovigilance

Pharmacovigilance is defined as "the science and activities relating to the detection, assessment, understanding and prevention of adverse effects or any drug-related problem" (3). It is important to note that this definition does not limit itself to the collection and evaluation of spontaneous case reports of suspected adverse drug reactions and includes pharmacoepidemiology studies (4). The role of a pharmaco-vigilance program is to identify signals that, upon further evaluation, lead to the discovery of previously "unknown" (meaning unidentified or unrecognized) or insufficiently understood adverse drug reactions that could not have been identified in the pre-approval period. Such adverse reactions can be due to previously unrecognized pharmacological effects of the drug, idiosyncratic (meaning unrecognized underlying mechanism) effects, drug-drug interactions, drug-food interactions, drug-disease interactions, factors related to specific patient populations, individual patient factors (such as pharmacogenomic factors), medication errors, or other factors such as being too infrequent to be identified in a few thousand patients. Ideally, a post-marketing safety surveillance system could identify these reactions rapidly and efficiently. After signal identification, an ideal drug safety system could determine the causal role of the drug, characterize the clinical spectrum of the adverse reaction, quantify the risk of the adverse reaction in a population treated with the drug, take appropriate regulatory action to prevent or minimize risk, and communicate these findings to healthcare professionals and patients.

c. Definition and taxonomy of drug safety signals

A number of definitions for the term "signal" have been proposed and there is considerable variation and ambiguity in its use in scientific publications, guidance documents and product information (5). A signal in pharmacovigilance was defined by WHO in 2002 as "Reported information on a possible causal relationship between an adverse event and a drug, the relationship being previously unknown or incompletely documented. Usually more than a single case report is required to generate a signal, depending on the seriousness of the event and quality of the information" (6). The CIOMS Working Group IV defined a signal as "A report or reports of an event with an unknown causal relationship to treatment that is recognized as worthy of further exploration and continued surveillance" (7).

Hauben and Aronson (8) provided a systematic review and lexicographic analysis of various definitions of signals in current use in pharmacovigilance and proposed a new definition. For purposes of this report, the following modification of this definition is used to define a signal:

"Information that arises from one or multiple sources (including observations and experiments), which suggests a new potentially causal association, or a new aspect of a known association, between an intervention and an event or set of related events, either adverse or beneficial, that is judged to be of sufficient likelihood to justify verificatory action."

14

The concept of "signal" requires an initial evaluation or clarification step to determine whether a particular case series ("messages" according to Hauben and Aronson), less frequently one single case, that has raised attention will require further evaluation. Once this first step has been completed, the safety finding becomes a signal which can either be "verified", "refuted" or remains "indeterminate".

To become a risk, a signal will require some reasonable knowledge of its probability of occurrence (see Glossary for a definition of risk). As such, an "indeterminate" signal goes hand in hand with a "potential risk", defined in the context of risk management as "an untoward occurrence in which there is some basis for suspicion of an association with the medicinal product of interest but where this association has not been confirmed" (9). Likewise, a "verified" signal would correspond to an "identified" risk. In this particular case, the association between an event and a drug has been confirmed and its likelihood of occurrence is reasonably established.

Examples include:

1. A reaction that is known to be associated with other products of the same class, or which could be expected to occur based on the properties of the medicinal product but which has never been observed so far in the pre- and post-approval setting with the drug under scrutiny (potential risk, not signal);

2. Cases of a designated medical event (DME) arising from a spontaneous adverse reaction reporting system (signal, potential risk);

3. Adverse reactions that have been observed in clinical trials or epidemiological studies for which the magnitude of the difference, compared with the comparator group (placebo or active substance, or unexposed group), on the parameter of interest is large enough to suggest a causal relationship (verified signal, identified risk).

Finally, a signal can be dismissed or refuted, in which case it likely represents a "false positive" that will return to the status of safety observation ("message") that may warrant further monitoring according to steps described in the signal detection process until new information arises that changes its status to "signal".

The taxonomy of drug safety signals is based on two distinct types of information:
1. Clinical signals are detected from noteworthy findings in individual case reports submitted either as solicited reports in active surveillance systems or unsolicited (spontaneous) reports in passive surveillance systems.

2. Statistical or quantitative signals are detected from group-level numerical differences in aggregate data from clinical trials, epidemiological studies (i.e. active surveillance systems); and spontaneous reports (in which numerical differences reflect the distribution of reported events for a given drug(s)).

Examples of clinical information detectable through the review of individual case reports that could represent a signal include:
- Rapid onset of an acute adverse event following exposure to a drug;
- "High quality" positive dechallenge/re-challenge (see Chapter VII for further discussion);

- Dose relationship;
- Three or more cases, say, of a rare adverse reaction that has a near-zero background incidence rate in the general population;
- Designated medical events (DMEs), such as agranulocytosis, that are known to be rare, serious and highly attributable to drugs.

Examples of statistical signals that may be detected by the analysis of aggregate data include:

- A statistically significant ($p<0.05$) higher rate of a serious adverse event (that was not a pre-specified endpoint) in the treatment group versus the comparator group in a single randomized controlled trial that conducted hundreds of multiple comparisons in analyzing its safety data;
- A consistent pattern of a numerically higher rate of a specific serious adverse event in the treatment group versus the comparator group across several randomized controlled trials included in a meta-analysis for which the p-value for the between-group comparison in any individual trial did not achieve statistical significance at the $p<0.05$ level;
- A statistically significant difference in the mean change from baseline versus the comparator group of a laboratory measure (e.g. liver transaminases) believed to be a biomarker for a future serious adverse drug reaction (e.g. acute liver failure) for which there was not a single case observed in the trial;
- A difference in the rate of an adverse reaction comparing the first month of follow-up after the start of treatment to the rate in the second to sixth month of follow-up in a prescription event monitoring study that conducted hundreds of multiple comparisons;
- A higher odds of prenatal exposure to a specific drug comparing mothers of children with a specific birth defect to mothers of healthy children in a case-control surveillance study that conducted hundreds of multiple comparisons;
- An increase in the incidence of a designated medical reaction (e.g. Guillain-Barré syndrome) in the general population in a population-based surveillance program (ecological study) comparing calendar periods before and after the introduction of a new vaccine.
- An "observed-to-expected" (O/E) ratio of spontaneous reporting frequency based on a 2x2 contingency table that cross-classifies and tabulates reports according to the presence or absence of a specific drug of interest and event of interest ("disproportionality analysis") that exceeds a pre-specified threshold of "interestingness".

d. Conclusions and recommendations

- Pharmacovigilance is an evolving discipline though its goals – to detect, assess, understand and prevent drug-related adverse effects – remain constant.

- The diversity of sources of information relevant to pharmacovigilance merit a definition of the term "signal" which is relevant to and encompasses these sources.

- The definition adopted for the purpose of this report includes reference to the diversity of sources information; goes further to include the concept of benefit as well as harm; and makes reference to the element of judgment that verificatory action is justified. This definition is based on a systematic review of various definitions in current use. It will need to be kept under review as the field of pharmacovigilance evolves.

- The confirmation of a risk as a consequence of detection of a signal requires careful consideration and a reasonable level of knowledge of its probability of occurrence. This may be a complex process and those involved need to be clear on the level of uncertainty as well as of knowledge.

References

1. Dieppe P, Bartlett C, Davey P et al. Balancing benefits and harms: the example of non-steroidal anti-inflammatory drugs. *British Medical Journal*, 2004, 329:31-34.

2. CIOMS Working Group VI. *Management of safety information from clinical trials*. Geneva, CIOMS, 2005: p. 31.

3. *The importance of pharmacovigilance – safety monitoring of medicinal products.* Geneva, WHO, 2002.

4. ICH E2E. *Harmonized tripartite guideline on pharmacovigilance planning,* 2004. (http://www.ich.org).

5. Hauben M, Reich L. Communication of findings in pharmacovigilance: use of the term signal and the need for precision in its use. *European Journal of Clinical Pharmacology,* 2005, 61(5-6):479-80.

6. *Safety of medicines: a guide to detecting and reporting adverse drug reactions.* Geneva, WHO, 2002. (http://whqlibdoc.who.int/hq/2002/WHO_EDM_QSM_2002.2.pdf).

7. CIOMS Working Group IV. *Benefit-risk balance for marketed drugs: evaluating safety signals.* Geneva, CIOMS, 1999: p. 95.

8. Hauben M, Aronson JK. Defining 'signal' and its subtypes in pharmacovigilance based on a systematic review of previous definitions. *Drug Safety,* 2009, 32(2):99-110.

9. EMEA/CHMP *Guideline on risk management systems for medicinal products for human use.* 20 November 2005.

III

Overview of approaches to signal detection

Monitoring the safety of medicinal products after licensure has historically been performed via spontaneous reporting systems (SRSs). These are passive public health surveillance systems that were put in place by different countries around the world in the 1960s, following the thalidomide tragedy. Although other approaches have been introduced with the goal of more proactive identification of hazards associated with the use of medicines after their initial authorisation, the role of SRSs remains very important (*1*).

The sources of pharmacovigilance information have been reviewed briefly in the Report of the CIOMS Working Group V (*2*) and in the ICH E2D guideline, "Post-approval safety data management" (definitions and standards for expedited reporting) (*3*) (see Table 1). In addition, electronic health/patient record or medical claim databases are being increasingly recognized as important sources of clinical safety data.

Table 1: Sources of clinical safety data during the post-approval phase described in the ICH E2D Guideline

Sources of individual case reports	Description of the source
I. Unsolicited sources	Spontaneous reports; Literature; Internet; Other sources (lay press or other media).
II. Solicited sources	Organised data collection systems (these include clinical trials, registries, post-approval named patient use programs, other patient support and disease management programs, surveys of patients or health care professionals, information gathering on efficacy or patient outcome; some of these may involve record-linkage, i.e. finding entries that refer to the same entity in two or more files).
III. Contractual agreements	Inter-company exchange of safety information.
IV. Regulatory authority sources	Individual Case Safety Reports, such as Suspected Unexpected Serious Adverse Reactions (SUSARs) that originate from regulatory authorities.

The range of organizations participating in the collection and analysis of pharmacovigilance data includes pharmaceutical companies, regulatory authorities, and national and international drug-monitoring centres. In addition, there are drug monitoring programs that are based at academic medical centres, e.g. the Research on

Adverse Drug events And Reports (RADAR) project (4), and specialized adverse event registries, such as the National Registry for Drug Induced Ocular Side Effects (5) in the USA, and the registry for severe skin reactions in Germany (Dokumentationszentrum schwerer Hautreaktionen, dZh) (6). Not all of these represent independent data sets (see Chapter V) and some individual reports may be present in more than one database. For example, the registries above are a reporting source for governmental and pharmaceutical company-sponsored SRSs.

In recent years, statistical methods for systematically sifting a large amount of SRS data have been developed (see Chapter VII). These tools and methods have collectively been termed "data mining". When considering the introduction of these new analytical approaches, an organization should place them, along with other existing methods ("traditional" pharmacovigilance approaches), in an integrated framework of a signal detection program (see also Chapter VIII).

a. Traditional approaches

Traditional pharmacovigilance methods for analysis of spontaneous adverse event reports include (7):

- Review of individual cases or case series in a pharmacovigilance database or in published medical or scientific literature; and

- Aggregate analyses of case reports using absolute case counts, simple reporting rates or exposure-adjusted reporting rates.

Traditional pharmacovigilance approaches are particularly important in the assessment of designated medical events (DMEs) or rare events for which clinical evaluation of individual cases tends to carry a larger weight and for which there may be an especially high premium on sensitivity over specificity. Detailed descriptions and discussions of spontaneous adverse event reports and qualitative methods of signal detection are provided in Chapters IV and VI respectively.

Once a signal is detected as a result of individual or aggregate analysis of spontaneous adverse event reports, it needs to be investigated through sequential steps, which include signal triage, clarification and early evaluation, and, if required, formal evaluation using independent data sets, such as hypothesis-testing research studies (see Chapter IX). Such investigation must be conducted in an integrated, holistic fashion within the context of biological plausibility and other available scientific evidence. The following data sources, although not necessarily used in all signal evaluations, should be considered for technical merit in providing useful additional information:

- Population-based databases (e.g. insurance claim or electronic patient record databases);

- Non-interventional (observational) studies (pharmacoepidemiological studies and patient registry studies);

- Knowledge regarding drugs in the same pharmacologic class;

- Background rates of the event under investigation in patients with relevant underlying disease conditions;

- Non-clinical and pharmacology studies;

- Mechanistic studies of the adverse effect;

- Clinical trials; and

- Industry data on product complaints.

b. Emergence of statistical data mining methods

Statistical data mining methods emerged in the late 1990s and complement traditional signal detection approaches in routine assessment of spontaneous adverse event report data (8, 9, 10, 11).

Statistical methods were originally developed as a means of performing systematic signal detection in large databases from the spontaneous reporting systems (SRSs) of adverse event information maintained by health authorities and drug monitoring centres; e.g. the WHO International Drug Monitoring program, the United States FDA Adverse Event Reporting System (AERS), the United Kingdom's Medicines Control Agency's ADROIT (now Sentinel) database, and EudraVigilance of the European Medicines Agency (EMA). These SRSs are characterized by the large numbers of adverse event reports, which are challenging to the capabilities of traditional pharmacovigilance approaches. The sheer volume and complexity of data represented in these large datasets, when only the traditional approaches are used, can increase the chances of not noticing early signals for some drug-induced ADRs, with significant public health impact.

Another characteristic of large SRSs maintained by health authorities and monitoring centres is the high degree of heterogeneity and diversity of individual drugs and drug classes represented, providing robust background (reference) data that are less likely to suffer from phenomena called "masking" or "cloaking" of drug-event associations, compared with smaller or less diverse databases, such as proprietary databases typically held by pharmaceutical companies. Despite these well-established limitations, pharmaceutical companies have been increasingly adopting statistical data mining as a component of a signal detection program in their proprietary spontaneous reporting databases, sometimes in parallel with data mining of health authority or drug monitoring centre databases.

Technical details of statistical data mining methods are described in Chapter VII. In appropriate settings, data mining may enhance the efficiency of a pharmacovigilance program by detecting some signals that would not otherwise be detected or would be detected substantially later if traditional approaches were used alone (although the converse may be true for other signals). Data mining methods generally identify drug-event combinations that are disproportional to pooled or overall distributions in the background dataset, which consists of a selection of all drug-event combinations. No causality can be inferred from the finding of disproportionality alone; rather, higher frequency of reporting than expected is highlighted for further evaluation including clinical review. The choice of the background dataset impacts the disproportionality analysis results; in particular, the size of the dataset and its heterogeneity with respect to the products (drugs) and the adverse events represented are critical factors.

c. Conceptual framework for integrating traditional and statistical data mining methods

A general framework of a typical signal detection program, that is, a flow of sequential steps of signal detection, prioritization, and evaluation as well as its linkage to risk management activities, is depicted in Figure 1. Data sources and analytical approaches in the signal evaluation step should be selected to suit the needs of a particular signal being assessed (e.g. not all signals would require a pharmacoepidemiological study).

Figure 1. Signal management process

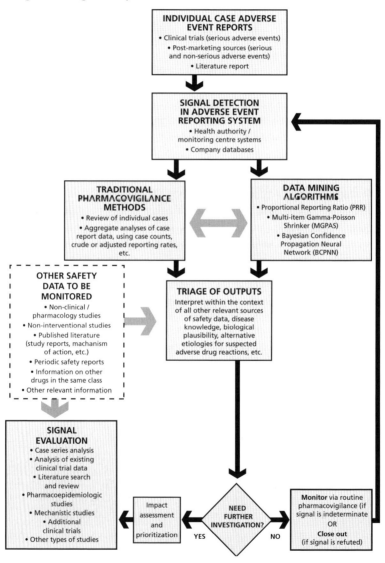

It should be noted that the addition of statistical data mining approaches does not necessarily change the overall framework and process flow of a signal detection program. Rather, those quantitative methods are intended to provide pharmacovigilance organisations with methods for systematically assessing spontaneous adverse event data that have been validated (*1, 2* in Chapter II).

Integration of statistical data mining approaches into a signal detection program requires appreciation of the strengths and limitations of data sources and statistical methods selected as well as adequate subject matter expertise in the application of data mining approaches. Points to consider when planning and implementing an integrated signal detection program involving data mining methods are described in Chapter VIII.

d. Interpretation of data mining results within an integrated approach

When applying disproportionality analysis, the known limitations of spontaneous adverse event reporting system should be recognized. Quantitative methods of signal detection cannot eliminate confounding by indication and other biases inherent in spontaneous adverse event report data, substantial deficits and distortions in the individual case-level data, or problems in the overall mechanism of data acquisition. Limitations of spontaneous report data, including data quality considerations, are discussed in more detail in Chapters IV and VIII respectively.

The critical aspect of the integration of statistical data mining methods alongside traditional methods of signal detection in pharmacovigilance is the scientific evaluation of the disproportionality analysis results. The interpretation of data mining outputs should take place within the context of other safety data derived from relevant sources (*12*); it should take into account the known safety profile and pharmacology of a medicinal product, knowledge of the patient populations being treated, biological plausibility, and alternative etiologies for suspected adverse drug reactions.

Selection of methodological specifications for disproportionality analysis (e.g. data sources, statistical methods, thresholds for filtering) and application of pharmacovigilance expertise and clinical judgment to the interpretation of disproportionality analysis results require a series of decisions. For this to take place in a systematic and reproducible fashion, an organization considering the adoption of disproportionality analysis data mining as a supplement to the traditional pharmacovigilance program should develop cohesive and transparent business practices (*13, 14*), which then should be reflected in standard operating procedures (SOPs), to support the integrated approach for the entire signal detection, evaluation, and management process (see Chapter IX). Adequate documentation of decisions and actions taken throughout the assessment of observations from disproportionality analysis is important to track signal detection activities and understand the evolution of emerging signals. A cross-functional team of qualified personnel, including drug safety scientists, epidemiologists, statisticians, data analysts, and physicians, is required for the interpretation and further evaluation of drug-event associations identified through quantitative signal detection.

e. Conclusions and recommendations

- Traditional pharmacovigilance approaches, based on spontaneous reporting systems, are particularly important in the assessment of rare events or designated medical events;

- Statistical methods for disproportionality analysis were originally developed as a means of performing systematic signal detection in large databases from the spontaneous reporting systems maintained by health authorities and drug monitoring centres, to complement traditional signal detection approaches;

- Integration of statistical data mining approaches does not necessarily change the overall framework and process flow of a signal detection program but requires appreciation of strengths and limitations of data sources and statistical methods selected and adequate subject matter expertise in application of data mining approaches;

- The interpretation of the outputs from disproportionality analysis should take place within the context of other safety data derived from relevant sources; and

- An organization considering the adoption of disproportionality analysis as a supplement to the traditional pharmacovigilance program should develop cohesive and transparent business practices reflected in standard operating procedures and should establish a cross-functional team of qualified personnel to ensure appropriate interpretation and management of the process outputs.

References

1. van Puijenbroek EP. Case reports and drug safety. *Drug Safety*, 2006, 29(8):643-5.

2. *Current challenges in pharmacovigilance: pragmatic approaches.* Report of CIOMS Working Group V. Geneva, CIOMS, 2001. ISBN 92 9036 074 7.

3. ICH E2D Guideline: *Post-approval safety data management: definitions and standards for expedited reporting.* Brussels, 2003. (http://www.ich.org/LOB/media/MEDIA631.pdf, accessed 19 August 2007).

4. Bennet CL et al. The research on adverse drug events and reports (RADAR) project. *Journal of the American Medical Association,* 2005, 293 (17):2131-2140.

5. Frauenfelder FW, Frauenfelder FT. Adverse ocular drug reactions recently identified by the national registry of drug-induced ocular side effects. *Ophthalmology,* 2004, 111:1275-1279.

6. http://www.uniklinik-freiburg.de/hautklinik/live/dzh.html (accessed 26 December 2007).

7. *Guidance for industry: good pharmacovigilance practices and pharmacoepidemiologic assessment.* US FDA, March 2005. (http://www.fda.gov/cder/guidance/6359OCC.htm).

8. Bate A, Lindquist M, Edwards IR et al. A Bayesian neural network method for adverse drug reaction signal generation. *European Journal of Clinical Pharmacology*, 1998, 54:315-21.

9. Evans SJW, Waller PC, Davis S. Use of proportional reporting ratios (PPRs) for signal generation from spontaneous adverse drug reaction reports. *Pharmacoepidemiol Drug Safety*, 2001, 10:483-6.

10. Szarman A, Machado SG, O'Neill RT. Use of screening algorithms and computer systems to efficiently signal higher-than-expected combinations of drugs and events in the US FDA'a spontaneous reports database. *Drug Safety*, 2002, 25 (6):381-92.

11. EudraVigilance Expert Working Group. *Guideline on the use of statistical signal detection methods in the EudraVigilance data analysis system.* London: European Medicines Agency; June 2008.

12. Almenoff J et al. Perspectives on the use of quantitative signal detection in pharmacovigilance. *Drug Safety*, 2005, 28(11):981-1007.

13. Waller PC, Heeley E, Moseley J. Impact analysis of signals detected from spontaneous adverse drug reaction reporting data. *Drug Safety,* 2005, 28(10):843-850.

14. Ståhl M et al. Introducing triage logic as a new strategy for the detection of signals in the WHO Drug Monitoring database. *Pharmacoepidemiology and Drug Safety,* 2004, 13:355-363.

IV

Spontaneously reported drug safety-related information

a. Definitions of adverse event and reaction

Critical to clear understanding and communication in pharmacovigilance is precise use of agreed definitions. The ICH E6 Guideline on Good Clinical Practice (*1*) defines an *adverse event* (AE) as "Any untoward medical occurrence in a patient or subject [in a clinical trial] administered a pharmaceutical product and which does not necessarily have a causal relationship with this treatment. An adverse event can therefore be any unfavorable and unintended sign (including an abnormal laboratory finding), symptom, or disease temporally associated with the use of a medicinal (investigational) product, whether or not related to the medicinal (investigational) product".

If the specific cause of an observed adverse event is not known, then it remains an unattributed adverse event. However, if a physician believes that there is a "reasonable possibility" that the adverse event may have occurred as a direct consequence of a medicinal product, then the adverse event becomes a *suspected adverse drug reaction* (suspected ADR). The definition of a suspected adverse drug reaction, incorporating the concept of "relatedness", is found in the ICH E2A Guidance (*2*), which states that a suspected adverse drug reaction is "A noxious and unintended response to any dose of a medicinal product for which there is a reasonable possibility that the product caused the response. In this definition, the phrase a "reasonable possibility" means that the relationship cannot be ruled out".

The conceptual distinction between 'adverse events', 'adverse drug reactions', 'suspected adverse drug reactions' and 'medication errors' has been described by Aronson and Ferner (*3*). Only 'adverse events' and 'suspected adverse drug reactions' can be observed and enumerated in practice. The actual numbers of adverse events that are true 'adverse drug reactions' cannot be determined with absolute certainty. In addition, the actual number of all spontaneous case reports of 'suspect adverse drug reactions' that are true 'adverse drug reactions' cannot be known with absolute certainty.

b. Data elements in a spontaneous reporting system

The data elements collected on spontaneous reports and entered into a database will determine the options for performing clinical and/or statistical assessment of adverse event reporting information, e.g. signal detection and evaluation.

A core set of standard data elements is harmonised at international level for electronic exchange of individual cases (ICH E2B(R2)); however, the specification for the use of certain data fields is not always consistent amongst various involved parties, particularly in different regulatory jurisdictions (4,5). The data, however, should be collected regardless of the nature of the adverse drug reaction experienced by the patient. The ICH E2B(R2)-specified data elements define the minimum dataset required for a valid report: (a) an identifiable patient, (b) an adverse event/reaction, (c) a suspect medicinal product, and (d) an identifiable reporter. However, it is widely recognised that the information required to perform an optimal scientific causality assessment can differ significantly according to the nature of the adverse reaction. These more specific data elements relate mainly to differential diagnoses to be considered by the reporter, which might exclude other (non-iatrogenic) causes of the reaction or might include expected events associated with underlying or pre-existing medical conditions. Attempts have been made in the past, in pharmacovigilance consensus fora, to identify the elements of information which are important to include in case reports and useful in the performance of causality assessment in specific situations (6), e.g. drug-induced liver reactions, drug-induced haematological reactions, drug-induced skin reactions, etc., but a universally agreed approach remains elusive. The presence of a case narrative containing all the information necessary to perform a causality assessment, which may not be consistently captured in the E2B(R2) structured data elements, e.g. time course of events, differential diagnoses considered by the reporter, etc., is still necessary to ensure the quality of the reports for signal evaluation (see ICH E2D and recommendations from the CIOMS Working Group V).

Relevant to this is that the method of collection of information for different SRSs may differ between systems that have been put in place by different organisations, e.g. regulatory authorities, national pharmacovigilance centres, or pharmaceutical companies. The information in spontaneous reports is sometimes collected either by direct communication with the reporter (e.g. healthcare professionals) or via the use of reporting forms which contain some standard elements of information, e.g. the United Kingdom Yellow Card scheme. In the case of direct communication with the healthcare professionals (HCP), the type of HCP collecting the information and the tool used (via targeted questionnaires or toxicity-specific forms) can influence the quality and level of data obtained. Some organisations prefer to customise the follow-up of selected information that may warrant further investigation (7) rather than collect information in an open-ended fashion. Little research has been performed to assess which is the more effective way of collecting initial or follow-up information in spontaneous reports, but some recommendations have been published by regulatory authorities.

The data elements collected via the report, the method of collection of the reports, the follow-up of initial reports, and the targeted search of information in specific situations etc., contribute to variability in the information collected on spontaneous reports and the results obtained from the traditional and quantitative methods that are applied to these reports. The implementation of the ICH E2B(R2) electronic standard in pharmacovigilance databases, with structured data elements, mitigates such variability and provides an excellent opportunity to extract more information with greater consistency than in the past, when pharmacovigilance databases were neither harmonised nor as exhaustive as they tend to be now. In the future, it may be possible to use consensus data standards and interoperability of computer systems to extract digitised safety data from Electronic Medical Records and transmit these data directly from the point of care to regulators and manufacturers. This could enhance both the quantity and quality of data available for timely signal detection activities.

c. Mechanisms for reporting

Collection and exchange of individual case safety reports has traditionally been on paper or by telephone. It is now technically feasible to use electronic means to collect and transmit safety data in support of improved signal detection. For example, collection of suspected adverse reactions directly from the point of patient care, i.e. from healthcare professionals, patients etc. can be accomplished via electronic means. Limited work has been done so far to assess their value in the context of signal detection. In 2007 the United Kingdom Medicines and Healthcare products Regulatory Agency (MHRA) implemented a direct electronic reporting scheme ("Yellow Card online") to encourage consumers and healthcare professionals to report suspected adverse reactions and suspected defects in medicinal products, as well as adverse incidents involving a medical device ("User reporting online") (8). The Netherlands Pharmacovigilance Centre Lareb provides electronic forms (Dutch language only) for healthcare professionals and patients to report suspected adverse reactions (9). The proportion of reports received by the Lareb direct reporting program in 2004, 2005, and 2006 was 11.7, 18.2, and 18.9 per cent of all reports (10). In 2008 Lareb received 7,414 reports from healthcare professionals, patients, authorization holders, and the National Vaccination Program. Patients were the source of 17.6% (n=1,304) of these reports. In the United States, reporting of adverse experiences following vaccination to the Vaccine Adverse Event Reporting System (VAERS) via the Internet became available to the public under a voluntary program in 2002. One early evaluation noted a somewhat better completion of such "web-reports" (11). The MHRA online form has automatically-applied electronic business rules to ensure that all necessary data fields are completed before the report is accepted and transmitted to the database.

Mandatory electronic safety reporting to competent authorities by marketing authorisation holders and sponsors of clinical trials of both expedited and non-expedited individual case safety reports (ICSRs) using ICH standards has been routine in Europe, Japan, and the United States for several years. Indeed, regulations require the electronic exchange of case reports from manufacturers to regulators and vice-versa in many regulatory jurisdictions (12). The experience gathered by the FDA/CDER using electronic standards to communicate with manufacturers in a voluntary program for marketed products demonstrated a dramatic reduction in data entry costs and also in the time taken to send an expedited report to a risk assessor (13). This improved business efficiency at the agency and permitted an enlightened allocation of available resources by shifting manpower from data entry activities to complementary pharmacovigilance activities, such as the interpretation of data. Between 1997 and 2009, the proportion of expedited ICSRs for marketed medicinal products voluntarily submitted to the FDA by manufacturers in electronic format gradually increased to over 84% of the total (*14*). The EMA has been actively exchanging electronic case data for both marketed products and from clinical trials since the EudraVigilance (*15*) database was placed in production with national competent authorities and marketing authorisation holders in 2001. Sponsors of clinical trials also submit expedited reports electronically to EudraVigilance over the Internet or via a web-based application. This provides a continuum of safety data over the lifecycle of a product, from first use in human studies through to maturation of the product in the market. Such electronic transmissions ensure high-fidelity transfer of data and support complete datasets that might otherwise lack the structured data that are required for robust analyses.

In summary, the increasing use of electronic safety reporting has facilitated a shift in relative focus from manual case handling/management to the scientific analysis of case-level and aggregate safety information, and facilitated the establishment of automated screening procedures.

d. Patient and consumer reporting

Patient and consumer reporting of adverse reactions has been implemented in several countries world-wide, including Australia, Canada, Denmark, the Netherlands, Sweden, the United Kingdom and the United States. A pilot with HIV-infected patients was begun in France in 2002. The advantages and disadvantages of direct patient reporting to medicines regulatory authorities have been identified and discussed in the literature (*16, 17, 18*). However, only limited work has been done to assess the impact of patient reporting on the detection of new signals in pharmacovigilance. This is currently an active area of research and in the near future the results of studies are expected on the value of patient reporting for signal detection.

Quality of patient compared to healthcare professionals reports

Despite the absence of agreed standards of data quality in pharmacovigilance, one pilot study conducted by the Netherlands Pharmacovigilance Centre Lareb between 2003 and 2004 following the introduction of a pilot phase of patient reporting, assessed the quality of the patients' reports compared to those received from healthcare professionals. The classification was based on the completeness of the reporting form submitted by patients. The study concluded that patient and healthcare professional reports were of similar quality, with 32% of the reports considered to be of good quality (*19*). However, differences in healthcare delivery/public health systems and privacy laws (which may impact on the feasibility of obtaining follow-up information) across regulatory jurisdictions account for substantial variability in the quality of patient/consumer reports.

Pattern of seriousness of patient reports

The same pilot study conducted by the Lareb showed that patients tended to report more serious adverse drug reactions than healthcare professionals. Twenty-nine percent of the patient reports (80) were considered to be serious, compared to 21% of those reported by the healthcare professionals (657). A subsequent longer-term study failed to show any difference; however, the two studies highlighted differences in the categories of seriousness.

Adverse reactions reported by patients tend to differ in content from those reported by healthcare professionals. Several studies suggest that by questioning the likelihood of a causal relationship between the drug and the occurrence of a reaction, physicians tend to filter the information reported by the patients on adverse drug reactions (even when the reaction is well established) (20). Patient reports received without the "filter" of healthcare professionals can highlight new adverse reactions and provide greater detail on known adverse reactions, particularly on the impact on quality of life. However, the terminology used by the patients is not always correctly understood by healthcare professionals. Furthermore this "filter" should not be seen as entirely detrimental as it might effectively filter out spurious associations.

Impact of patient reports on timing

The timeliness of information acquisition and the quality of that information are crucial determinants of the value of patient reports for improving the safety monitoring of medicines and public health protection. Several studies reported favourably on direct reporting by patients, noting that they tend to notify about adverse drug events earlier than healthcare workers (21). Since patients and their non-healthcare professional caregivers are often the first to recognise an adverse reaction, particularly in non-hospital settings, it follows that they would be in a position to report adverse reactions sooner than healthcare professionals. Patients and consumers should be encouraged to consult with their healthcare provider as soon as an adverse reaction is suspected.

Volume of patient reports

One concern about patient reporting has been the potential for pharmacovigilance systems to be overwhelmed with reports of minor symptoms and cases where the patient is unable to discriminate effectively between symptoms attributable to individual drugs or diseases. These factors could exacerbate the challenge of identifying true signals in the background noise of patient reports. In a methodological study in the United Kingdom, patients receiving one of nine drugs under intensive monitoring were surveyed regarding adverse drug reactions. The results suggested that only 54% of patients reported some or all of their symptoms to their doctor; a case-note review of a sample of these patients found that only 22% were recorded by the doctor and just 0.4% of all symptoms were reported to the United Kingdom Committee on Safety of Medicines (22). It can, therefore, be expected that provision for direct reporting of adverse drug reactions by patients will increase the volume of available reports.

However, studies published on patient reporting of adverse reactions showed that patients' reports comprised less than 10% of total reports. A recent study describing the long term experience of patient reporting in the Netherlands showed an increase in patient reports to approximately 20% of the total number received over a three-year period (April 2004 until April 2007). This increase is consistent with the increase in number (and respective percentage) of reports from consumers received by the United

States FDA in AERS. Between 1998 and 2007, the absolute number and proportion of consumer reports received in AERS increased from approximately 24,000 to approximately 175,000, and from 22% to 46% of the total cases received annually in AERS (*23*).

Patient (and healthcare professional) reporting can be stimulated by news in the mass media, e.g. the measles-mumps-rubella vaccine and autism debate in the United Kingdom and the United States; such reports can result in a biased over-representation of reports for certain event types in an SRS database. Furthermore, when reports are accepted directly from patients, the possibility exists that spurious reports could be processed as a result of consumer dissatisfaction, litigation or devious counter-detailing by rogue competitors. Such occurrences could skew the results of automated signal detection.

In conclusion, although limited work has been published on patient reporting of adverse drug reactions and the application of signal detection methodologies to such data, and some of this limited work may have significant methodological limitations, patient reporting may provide information on new adverse drug reactions earlier than when reported by healthcare professionals and new information on established adverse reactions, and there were no substantial differences in terms of data quality between patient reports and reports from healthcare professionals (the criteria used to assess the quality of the reports are not always explicit). Finally, the volume of reports from patients has increased substantially over the past 10 years.

e. Limitations and challenges of spontaneous data

Spontaneous adverse event data suffers from a number of well known limitations – under-reporting, the lack of exposure data – and biases, such as stimulated reporting (*24*).

It is recognised that data gathered from these sources cannot be used to quantify the extent of risk. Normally, spontaneous data can only supply a hypothesis that should be substantiated or possibly confirmed by other methods, such as clinical trials and observational studies. Nevertheless, studies on the publicly-available information underpinning decisions to withdraw medicinal products from the market show that spontaneous reports still play a major role in these decisions. This is a common scenario in pharmacovigilance, namely decision-making in the setting of residual uncertainty. These studies, conducted between 1999 and 2004, showed that case reports were the only evidence used in the withdrawal of a drug in 36% to 50% of drug-associated safety issues (*25, 26, 27, 28*).

Pharmacovigilance data sources can be classified as numerator-only (these include spontaneous reports and reports from literature) and numerator-plus-denominator sources (clinical trial data, electronic medical records). This distinction relates to the ability of these methods to identify, characterize, and/or quantify the level of risk associated with the administration of a medicine (incidence/prevalence) within a defined population and to help establish a causal relationship between the administration of the medicine and the occurrence of the events with varying degrees of certainty.

The identification of new safety signals arising from numerator/denominator-based methods of collection of safety data (including clinical trials) is complex and has been discussed in several articles and textbooks (*29, 30*). Although there is less experience using this method than with using SRS data, emergent research in numerator/denominator-based methods has identified these methods as major areas of interest. The CIOMS Working Group VI has published guidelines on the management of safety information arising from (interventional) clinical trials. Some attempts have been made to extend certain data-mining techniques to databases holding data obtained using these methods of collection.

Monitoring adverse events (AEs) via SRSs is practically challenging due to the need to reconcile a large number of individual initial and follow-up reports, and scientifically challenging due to the broad variety of medical conditions under surveillance. Reported AEs are both qualitatively and quantitatively diverse, and appreciating this helps in formulating signal detection and evaluation strategies. AEs may include clinical signs, symptoms, and syndromes that the non-specialist may not immediately recognize as potentially drug-related. In an SRS database, this variety of medical concepts is constantly increasing over time with the addition of novel therapies and the corresponding increase in molecular targets. The diversity in relative quantitative representation of the monitored events in exposed versus unexposed patients has practical implications for signal detection and evaluation. Table 2 provides insights into the quantitative variability that must be addressed in pharmacovigilance. Although the table, adapted from Aronson et al. (*31*), is geared to discussing the implications for confirming associations, the categories presented in the table deepen our understanding of the "sample space" of events and, therefore, has implications for initial signal detection as well.

Table 2: Quantitative characteristics of adverse event

Attributable incidence in patients taking drug	Background incidence of the event	Example	Ease of proving the association (method)
Common	Rare	Phocomelia due to thalidomide	Easy (clinical observation)
Rare	Rare	Aspirin (acetylsalicylic acid) and Reye's syndrome	Less easy (clinical observation)
Common	Common	Angiotensin Converting Enzyme inhibitors and cough	Difficult (large observational study)
Uncommon	Common to rare	Hormone Replacement Therapy and breast carcinoma	Very difficult (large clinical trial)
Rare	Common	None known	Virtually impossible

The practical implication of this clinical and quantitative diversity is that optimum signal detection requires the use of multiple methods and data streams and the avoidance of over-reliance on a single approach (*32*).

f. Reporting in special populations

Spontaneous reporting systems (SRS) databases and periodic aggregate reporting, e.g. periodic safety update reports (PSURs), can be used to monitor the safety of medicines in special populations. Quantitative methods may have a role in such monitoring, since it is technically possible to incorporate signalling mechanisms that relate to such special populations. For example, it is feasible to conduct focused signal detection in narrow age groups, e.g. children, adolescents, elderly people, and to subset the data for analysis accordingly. There is, currently, little experience in this regard and the generally limited amount of key covariates contained in SRS data place significant constraints on useful stratification options. Furthermore, the beneficial versus adverse effects of stratification in the context of quantitative methods of signal detection are still the subject of debate (*33, 34, 35*). Similarly, for periodic reporting of aggregate data, it is recommended that pharmacovigilance data be correlated with usage information according to age groups. More specifically, in the use of paediatric medicines, general as well as more specific pharmacovigilance guidance has been released in the United States and the European Union.

Whether included in the same or separate databases, signal detection in the specific case of vaccines requires special attention. However, a detailed description of these nuances is outside the scope of this report. As with the spontaneous reporting of safety information for medicinal products, it has been established that not all quantitative methods are useful in performing signal detection for vaccines and that the clinical significance of statistical performance gradients between methods is unclear (*36*). More active methods of surveillance are being developed for vaccine safety monitoring.

In the case of congenital malformations, additional methodologies can be applied, such as birth registries, which can be used for signal detection.

g. Conclusions and recommendations

- The spontaneous reporting systems remain an important source of signals and safety information once a drug is placed on the market. However, the data from spontaneous reporting suffer from important biases and limitations. These limitations must be kept in mind when interpreting the results of signal detection algorithms.

- Universally understood and accepted definitions of adverse event and reaction, suspected adverse reaction and medication error are critical to effective communication and research in pharmacovigilance.

- Internationally harmonised standards of spontaneous data transmission have enabled rapid transmission and exchange of data, and support ongoing developments of tools and methodologies to support better analysis.

- Patient and consumer reporting have been introduced widely and studies so far are encouraging in terms of data quality and timeliness. The patterns of reactions reported by patients and health care professionals are different (type of events, seriousness, temporality or timing of reporting). Further research is required on its value for signal detection.

- The well known limitations of spontaneous data support investigation of strategies to conduct signal detection using numerator plus denominator data. However, such strategies should not overlook the inherent value of the reporter's suspicion and deductive logic.

References

1. ICH E6 (R1). *Guideline on good clinical practice.* Current step 4 version dated 10 June 1996 (http://www.ich.org).

2. ICH E2A. *Guideline for industry: clinical safety data management: definitions and standards for expedited reporting.* Step 5 as of October 1994 (http://www.ich.org).

3. Aronson JK, Ferner RE. Clarification of terminology in drug safety. *Drug Safety*, 2005, 28:851-870.

4. ICH E2A *Guideline: Clinical safety data management. Definitions and standards for expedited reporting.* (http://www.ich.org/LOB/media/MEDIA436.pdf, accessed 19 August 2007).

5. ICH E2B *Guideline (renamed E2B(R2) Guideline in 2005): Maintenance of the clinical safety data management guideline including data elements for transmission of individual case safety reports.* 1997. (http://www.ich.org/LOB/media/MEDIA2217.pdf, accessed 19 August 2007).

6. See for example, *Adverse drug reactions. A practical guide to diagnosis and management.* Chichester, UK, John Wiley & Sons, 1994. ISBN 0 471 94211 1.

7. US Department of Health and Human Services. Food and Drug Administration. *Guidance for industry. Good pharmacovigilance practices and pharmacoepidemiologic assessment.* March 2005. (http://www.fda.gov/CDER/guidance/6359OCC.pdf, accessed 19 August 2007).

8. MHRA online safety reporting for medicinal products, medical devices, and blood or blood components. (http://www.mhra.gov.uk/home/idcplg?IdcService=SS_GET_PAGE&nodeId=291, accessed 27 December 2007).

9. Lareb online reporting form (http://www.lareb.nl/melden/index.asp, accessed 27 December 2007).

10. Lareb safety monitoring annual reports with summary information on direct reporting (Dutch and English) (http://www.lareb.nl/documents/jaarverslag2006.pdf, accessed 27 December 2007).

11. Haber P, et al. Web-based reporting: 10 months experience in the vaccines adverse event reporting system (VAERS), USA; *Pharmacoepidemiology and Drug Safety*, vol 12; S46 (ICPE conf abstract).

12. *Volume 9A of the rules governing medicinal products in the European Union: pharmacovigilance for medicinal products for human use.* January 2007. (http://ec.europa.eu/enterprise/pharmaceuticals/eudralex/homev9.htm, accessed 19 August 2007).

13. CDER 2005 *Report to the nation – improving public health through human drugs.* (http://www.fda.gov/cder/reports/rtn/2005/rtn2005.pdf, accessed 27 December 2007).

14. Personal communication, Roger Goetsch, 10 October 2007.

15. Descriptive information on EudraVigilance. (http://eudravigilance.emea.europa.eu/human/EVBackground(FAQ).asp, accessed 27 December 2007).

16. Blenkinsopp A et al. Patient reporting of suspected adverse drug reactions: a review of published literature and international experience. *British Journal of Clinical Pharmacology*, 2006, 63(2):148-156.

17. See *Evaluation of patient reporting to the yellow card scheme, April 2006. Patient reporting of suspected adverse reactions*, document published by the MHRA.

(http://www.mhra.gov.uk/home/idcplg?IdcService=SS_GET_PAGE&nodeId=755, accessed 19 August 2007).

18. Effets indésirables: la notification directe par les patients est utile. *Prescrire*, 2004; 24(253):621-622.

19. van Grootheest AC, Passier JL, van Puijenbroek EP. Direct reporting of side effects by the patient: favourable experience in the first year. *Ned Tijdschr Geneeskd*, 2005, 149:529–533.

20. Golomb BA et al. Physician response to patient reports of adverse drug effects. Implications for patient-targeted adverse effect surveillance. *Drug Safety,* 2007; 30(8):669-675.

21. Egberts TCG et al. Can adverse drug reactions be detected earlier? A comparison of reports by patients and professionals. *British Medical Journal*, 1996, 313:530-531.

22. Jarernsiripornkul et al. Patient reporting of potential adverse drug reactions: a methodological study. *British Journal of Pharmacology*, 2002, 53:318-335.

23. http://www.fda.gov/cder/aers/statistics/aers_hcp_consumer.htm

24. Wise L et al. New approaches to drug safety: a pharmacovigilance tool kit. *Nature Reviews Drug Discovery*, 2009, 10:779-782.

25. Clarke A et al. An assessment of the publicly disseminated evidence of safety used in decisions to withdraw medicinal products from the UK and US markets. *Drug Safety*, 2006, 29(2):175-181.

26. Olivier P et al. The nature of scientific evidence leading to drug withdrawals for pharmacovigilance reasons in France. *Pharmacoepidemiology and Drug Safety*, 2006, 15(11):808-812.

27. Wysowski DK, Swartz L. Adverse drug event surveillance and drug withdrawals in the United States, 1969-2002: The importance of reporting suspected adverse reactions. *Archives of Internal Medicine*, 2005, 165:1363-1369.

28. Kuehn BM. FDA panel seeks to balance risks in warnings for antidepressants. *Journal of the American Medical Association*, 2007, 297(6):573-574.

29. Mann R, Andrews E, eds. *Pharmacovigilance.* Chichester, UK, John Wiley & Sons, 2002. ISBN 0 470 49441 0.

30. *Stephen's detection of new adverse drug reactions.* 5th ed. Talbot J, Waller P (eds). Chichester, UK, John Wiley & Sons, 2004. ISBN 0 470 54552 X.

31. Aronson JK, Ferner RE. Clarification of terminology in drug safety. *Drug Safety*, 2005, 28(10):851-70.

32. Hauben M. Signal detection in the pharmaceutical industry integrating clinical and computational approaches. *Drug Safety*, 2007, 30(7):627-630.

33. Hopstadius J et al. Impact of stratification on adverse event surveillance. *Drug Safety*, 2008, 31(11):1035-48.

34. Evans S. Stratification for spontaneous report databases. *Drug Safety*, 2008, 31(11):1049-52.

35. Hopstadius J et al. Stratification for spontaneous report databases. *Drug Safety, 2008, 31(12):1145-47.*

36. Banks D et al. Comparing data mining methods on the VAERS database. *Pharmacoepidemiology and Drug Safety*, 2005; 14(9):601-609.

V

Databases that support signal detection

The types of databases in existence which can be used for signal detection are presented in Table 3 which serves as a reference summary and basis for the discussion in this section. Appendix 3 provides a list of international and national spontaneous reporting systems (SRS) databases. While certain SRS data sets are publicly available, most are not. Redacted data, i.e. data with personal identifiers etc. rendered unreadable, from the FDA's AERS and the MHRA's Sentinel, for example, are available for public use.

Table 3: Databases that can be used for signal detection in the post-authorization period

Types of databases	Examples	Advantages	Disadvantages
Spontaneous Reporting System (SRS) databases	Vigibase (WHO), Eudra-Vigilance (EEA), AERS (US), Sentinel (UK)	National or regional in scope, high sensitivity in detecting rare AEs, relatively inexpensive	Requires reporter recognition Differential/biased reporting (e.g. underreporting, or in some cases stimulated/over-reporting, no denominator)
Prescription Event Monitoring databases	Drug Safety Research Unit (UK), the Intensive Medicines Monitoring Programme (New Zealand)	Systematic prospective targeted collection of detailed AE information via questionnaires to prescribers	Small size of cohort, limited information on risk factors, low response rate bias, no routine follow up, no good comparison group, resource-intensive (expensive)
Large linked administrative databases	Health care databases comprising automated administrative claims (e.g. in the US these are managed by for-profit Managed Care Organizations, or, in case of Medicare and Medicaid, sponsored by government)	Large population of patients; relatively long exposure; incidence rates in exposed and background rates of events can be calculated	Incompletely captured medical information; uninsured population not represented; data have been mainly used for observational studies – little experience of use in data mining; real time access to data difficult – for true prospective monitoring for targeted events; full access to data expensive
Electronic Medical Records (EMR) Databases	General Practice Research Database (UK)	More complete and longitudinal patient information, including various covariates (e.g. BMI), and risk factors (smoking, alcohol use, etc.)	Mainly used for observational studies – little experience of use in data mining; real time access to data difficult; expensive

a. Spontaneous reporting databases

The World Health Organization's Uppsala Monitoring Centre and regulatory authorities have developed pharmacovigilance databases that share some common features; most have been created to support national spontaneous reporting schemes. Some of the databases have been extensively modified to comply with ICH standards and requirements, including changes to medical terminology via implementation of the Medical Dictionary for Regulatory Activities (MedDRA). The volume of reports contained in the databases varies from several thousand to over four million. The type and range of medicinal products represented and the pattern of the background information held are variable and depend, in part, on the date the particular database was created and any subsequent enhancements; some contain reports going as far back as the early 1960s. Two well-known SRS databases are exclusively dedicated to the pharmacovigilance of vaccines (VAERS in the USA and CAEFISS in Canada). In addition, electronic exchange of Suspected Unexpected Serious Adverse Reaction reports (SUSARs) from interventional clinical trials is supported by some systems, e.g. EMA's EudraVigilance Clinical Trials Module and the system used by the Pharmaceutical and Medical Devices Agency (Japan).

The volume of reports and the type of products handled by the organisation need to be carefully considered as they will guide selection of the methods used to perform signal detection activities. It is widely acknowledged that certain traditional methods of signal detection may be advantageous when a low number of well documented cases are available to perform signal detection and for events for which a relative premium is placed on sensitivity over specificity. On the other hand, traditional quantative methods and data mining algorithms are more suitable to perform systematic, automated screening of large datasets (*1*) for conspicuous statistical associations.

Similarly, the characteristics of target product(s) can also influence the outputs of quantitative signal detection methods, since the products and their indications for use will determine the type of background information present in the pharmacovigilance database. This is the internal control against which the disproportionality analyses are conducted. In some instances, this background information may lead to a masking effect for certain events in disproportionality analysis, e.g. high representation of a particular class of products and/or an adverse event. This is particularly applicable to companies' proprietary SRS databases, which are generally less diverse than regulatory authorities' or monitoring centres' databases. However, since there is insufficient knowledge and experience to understand the net effect on performance characteristics of removing subsets of the databases for general signal detection purposes, it cannot be recommended as a routine procedure at this time.

In addition, the profile of medicines and spontaneous-sourced ICSRs reported with medicines in general has changed over the past decade. For example, an increasing number of spontaneous reports received in SRS databases involve biological medicinal products, which are produced by recombinant DNA technology, and antiretroviral agents, which are indicated for use in patients with long-term or progressive disease (*2*).

Advantages and limitations of spontaneous reporting databases

The advantages and limitations of these different SRS databases must be borne in mind when interpreting the statistics of disproportionate reporting. Database design features, which have varied from system to system over time, will have a critical influence on the background data encountered in any disproportionality analyses. The older databases, e.g. Vigibase or AERS, contain structured ICSR data for a wide range of products, including those which are no longer authorised, no longer marketed by the innovator, or simply no longer available, whereas newer products may be over-represented in more recently designed databases such as EudraVigilance. Antiretrovirals are over-represented in the French national database. This difference in background information may be pertinent to the detection of new signals for innovative products. Some databases contain spontaneous reports from patients, e.g. AERS, VAERS, Lareb, and MHRA's Sentinel (see Chapter IV, section e). Some databases contain little or no information on products in certain therapeutic categories. For example, AERS and Vigibase contain very few adverse event reports on vaccines. Therefore, the detection of new signals for this particular class of products using these databases may not be feasible at present. A pilot study in the United Kingdom compared signals detected on the national Sentinel database with those detected by Marketing Authorisation holders (3). This study found that different signals were detected from different databases over the same time-period.

b. Other datasets that can be used for signal detection

In addition to SRS databases, other data sources that provide information on patient exposure to medicinal products and medical outcomes can be considered for signal detection.

Cohort event monitoring

Cohort Event Monitoring (CEM) is a non-interventional method of intensive monitoring of newly marketed medicines. CEM collects data on cohorts of 10,000-12,000 users of new medicines via surveys of prescribers in New Zealand (by the Intensive Medicines Monitoring Programme (IMMP) and in the United Kingdom by the Drug Safety Research Unit (DSRU) at the University of Southampton (4, 5, 6).

Essentially, CEM assembles cohorts of consecutive drug users often by prescription registration (hence the alternative descriptor Prescription Event Monitoring – PEM). Once the method for assembling the cohort of exposed individuals is in place, health professionals are asked to report events, not suspected reactions, on a regular basis (IMMP), or to respond to specific questionnaires (IMMP and DSRU). The IMMP receives adverse event reports from all health care practitioners and patients. These reports are continuously analysed for new signals, and guide the design of questionnaires to health professionals or patients to gain further information. The DSRU does not regularly monitor the signals detected for confirmation by other datasets. In the pre-study phase, potential safety issues and available data on the safety profile are explored for tailoring of the study protocol. Also, after completion of a study, the data may be re-examined for evaluation of novel signals for the compound.

The CEM method has important strengths. The IMMP collects information on all patients exposed to the target drug, whilst the DSRU information is collected from a representative national sample of GPs. In both instances the information gained is from "real-world" situations. Prescription data are derived from prescriptions that are actually dispensed. The complete medical outcome information is gathered from GPs regardless of their assessment of causality/relatedness to the drug. Close contact between CEM researchers and GPs facilitates the follow-up of important events, pregnancies, and deaths. There are also some limitations that merit consideration when interpreting results from CEM. These include:

- Possible underreporting;

- The possibility for incomplete recording of patient data and the lack of prescription history in hospital settings;

- The relatively small size (10,000-15,000 persons) for detection of rare events; and

- The lack of naïve control groups. Cohorts of patients who have been or are monitored for other treatments have been used.

Two main types of signal detection methods have been used on CEM data: qualitative and quantitative (7). Similar to traditional manual methods employed in SRS, the qualitative method in CEM relies on astute clinicians/reviewers to evaluate information on individual cases, aiming at identifying clues of causality. Such assessments, when done on a case series of patient reports, take into consideration a number of facts such as time to onset information, biological and pharmacological plausibility based on knowledge of the drug, the possible effects of concomitant medicines, the role of underlying illness or co-morbidity, re-challenge and de-challenge information, etc. Researchers at the DSRU have applied the Bradford Hill criteria in the evaluation of potential signals (8).

A quantitative approach applied to CEM data involves analysis of Incidence Density (ID) rates. Typically, drug-event ID rates in the first month of exposure (DI1) are calculated and compared with the corresponding ID rates in the subsequent five months (DI2). Events are then ranked using ID difference value (DI1-DI2). IMMP approaches the quantification differently: there are annual questionnaires to the prescribing doctors asking them to examine their patients' records for new events occurring in a stated time period after the first prescription of the medicine and to compare with a similar time period before.

Since 2000, with the introduction of a new computer system, DSRU has been exploring the application of signal detection techniques using disproportionality analyses. As the DSRU database is large, with more than a million completed "Green Form" reports from more than 80 completed studies for various drugs, it theoretically allows for automated screening for statistics of disproportionate reporting. However, at present DSRU researchers have concluded that automated disproportionality methods add limited benefit when used on the PEM database, as most signals are detected manually due to heightened vigilance and the intensity of monitoring (9). The IMMP is also examining the use of disproportionality measures as well as the use of other ways of capturing their cohorts than by reviewing prescriptions.

c. Data quality

In pharmacovigilance, it is acknowledged that the interpretation of results from signal detection activities relies heavily on the quality of the information held on the database. This is particularly important for quantitative methods of signal detection, since these techniques homogenize spontaneous reports of variable quality and completeness, and provide numerical output devoid of clinical context.

A major limitation of spontaneous databases is the volume of duplicates, linked to the increased transmission of ICSRs relating to the same adverse event by different stakeholders (*10*).

Many large SRS databases contain duplicate reports, i.e. reports from different sources on the same adverse event in the same patient. For example, duplicate reports are present in AERS, Vigibase, and EudraVigilance. The identification and elimination of duplicates from analyses will, therefore, be advantageous for any signal evaluation. However, current duplicate detection procedures, some of which are applied prospectively (i.e. prior to data mining) and others retrospectively (i.e. after data mining), have limitations (see ref *10*) and enhanced methods of duplicate detection are being developed (*11*).

Data quality and pre-processing are important concerns and they may significantly influence the results of signal detection methods (*12*). In that respect, ICH E2B(R2)-compliant databases or those SRS databases which capture a case narrative will have an advantage over those that do not. Older reports may not be adequately documented or their data may not be adequately classified and structured in the database to perform a thorough signal assessment. Most modern databases have been designed to be in accordance with data elements specified in the ICH E2B(R2) standard. However, coding conventions, mapping of data elements from one system to another or migration of "older generation" data to a "newer generation" database may present challenges that must be considered when applying signal detection methods.

d. Pharmacoepidemiology resources

An informal list of resources prepared by members of the International Society of Pharmacoepidemiology (ISPE) in 2005 includes the names of various databases/ data collection systems that have been used in observational epidemiological and pharmacoepidemiological research. A modified version of this list (database resources stratified by country) is provided in Appendix 3, Table 2, of this report.

The following are major types of databases:
- National/provincial health care system databases (GPRD in the United Kingdom, Medicare/Medicaid/Veterans Administration in the United States);
- Medical insurance claims databases (United HealthCare, Medstat, Pharmetrics, etc.);
- Managed care organizations administrative databases (HMO research network);

- Electronic healthcare/medical records databases (GEMS, Cerner, etc.); and
- Survey/registry databases, national and regional (Prescription Event Monitoring, Slone cancer registry, etc.).

Details on most of these administrative data collection systems can be found on the corresponding web sites or in pharmacoepidemiology textbooks (*13*, *14*).

e. Conclusions and recommendations

- National and international databases which support signal detection vary considerably in size, structure and content. The special characteristics of the data held in a database need to be carefully taken into account when considering the application of signal detection methodologies. Research is needed to elucidate the impact of the various factors of size, product range and duration of existence on signal detection.

- A key issue for SRS databases is data quality, including the extent of duplicate reports in particular as the reporter base has extended to include patient and consumer reports.

- In addition to the spontaneous reporting databases, some other datasets (observational or active surveillance) can be used for signal detection purposes. These databases also require some extensive data management or manipulation, and may also suffer from strengths or limitations which must be considered during their use; the example of prescription event monitoring (PEM) illustrates the advantages and weaknesses of such active surveillance methods.

- Some datasets are publicly available although data are subject to redaction to protect privacy. The availability of different datasets has not, to date, been formally utilized and this needs to be further investigated.

- Future initiatives in different regions of the world are aimed in particular at setting up active surveillance networks which will play a major role in the future in signal detection and evaluation.

References

1. Almenoff J et al. Perspectives on the use of data mining in pharmacovigilance. *Drug Safety*, 2005, 28(11):981–1007.

2. Thiessard F et al. Trends in spontaneous adverse drug reaction reports to the French pharmacovigilance system (1986-2001). *Drug Safety*, 2005, 28(8):731-740.

3. Swain E et al. Early communication of drug safety concerns. *Pharmacoepidemiology and Drug Safety*, 2009. (www.interscience.wiley.com) DOI:10.1002/pds.1898.

4. Shakir SAW. Prescription Event Monitoring in Strom BL et al. *Pharmacoepidemiology* 4th edition. Chichester, UK, John Wiley & Sons. 2005. ISBN-10 0-470-86681-0.

5. Shakir SAW. PEM in the UK in Mann R and Andrews E et al. *Pharmacovigilance*. Chichester, UK, John Wiley & Sons. 2002. ISBN 0-470-49441-0.

6. Coulter DM. PEM in New-Zealand in Mann R and Andrews E et al. *Pharmacovigilance*. Chichester, UK, John Wiley & Sons. 2002. ISBN 0-470-49441-0.

7. Ferreira G. Prescription-event monitoring: developments in signal detection. *Drug Safety*, 2007, 30(7):639-41.

8. Perrio M, Voss S, Shakir SAW. Application of the Austin Bradford Hill criteria to assess causality in pharmacovigilance using the example of cisapride-induced arrhythmia. *Drug Safety*, 2006, 29(10):911-1010.

9. Shakir SAW. Thoughts on signal detection in pharmacovigilance. *Drug Safety*, 2007, 30(7):603-606.

10. Hauben M et al. Extreme duplication in the US FDA adverse events reporting system database. *Drug Safety*, 2007, 30(6):551-54.

11. Norén N, Bate A. A hit-miss model for duplicate detection in the WHO drug safety data base. Proc 11th ACM SIGKDD Int Conf Knowl Disc Data Mining. 2005:459-468. ISBN 1-59593-135-X.

12. Hauben M et al. Illusions of objectivity and a recommendation for reporting data mining results. *European Journal of Clinical Pharmacology*, 2007, 63(5):517-21.

13. See Automated data systems available for pharmacoepidemiology studies in Strom BL et al. *Pharmacoepidemiology,* 4th edition. Chichester, UK, John Wiley & Sons. 2005. ISBN-10 0-470-86681-0.

14. Mann R et al. *Part II signal generation in pharmacovigilance*. Chichester, UK, John Wiley & Sons. 2002. ISBN 0-470-49441-0.

VI

Traditional methods of signal detection

The methods of signal detection applied within an operational framework of a spontaneous reporting system may be broadly classified into two types: qualitative and quantitative. From a historical perspective, they may be roughly categorized as traditional versus enhanced quantitative, statistical or automated signal detection methods. Traditional methods include both qualitative (e.g. manual medical review of individual cases or case series) and simple quantitative approaches (e.g. frequency/reporting rates, sorting, cross-tabulation etc.). They have been long used in pharmacovigilance prior to the late 1990s, when a renaissance in statistical approaches occurred, in part as a consequence of the ever increasing volumes of spontaneous reports received and size of databases. In 1999, Amery listed several signalling methods (referred to as seven signal generation tools) for spontaneous adverse event reports (*1*). In their 2001 review, Clark and colleagues offered an alternative classification of published approaches to signal detection (*2, 3*). They described 11 groups of signalling methods based on signalling step and according to data analysis strategy.

a. Case and case series review

The "index case" or "striking case" method is probably the most commonly used technique in traditional pharmacovigilance. Trained product safety specialists detect signals while routinely reviewing submitted information, often during the initial intake assessment of individual case reports (spontaneous AE reports, AE reports from systematic data collection schemes, or cases published in the literature). The identification of even one well-documented ICSR with an unusual "striking" feature can sometime be interpreted as a signal, even though in practice, in most situations, strong suspicions about possible drug-event associations are usually based on a series of cases with similar reported features (clustering). Admittedly, such manual reviews are subjective and benefit from a thorough familiarity of the reviewer with the product pharmacology and the condition(s) for which it is indicated.

The relative contribution of individual case intake assessments and subsequent case series to the total number of signals detected is likely to be highly situation dependent. It may be very variable across organizations and, within an organization, across products and product life cycles. In some instances, the pertinent information may be related to the potential public health impact of the event on public safety and/or impact on the overall benefit-risk profile of the drug. Such circumstances may warrant placing a premium on sensitivity over specificity (*4*). It may be due to the clinical nature of the event itself, which may strongly suggest a credible relationship to the drug. Other features may be influential in concluding that a signal of suspected causality is present. For example, positive de-challenge/re-challenge may be used to move an association to the designation of a signal in some instances. For the latter, it is important to note that reported de-challenge and re-challenge may carry more or less evidentiary weight depending on specific characteristics, such as whether the rechallenge is blinded, accompanied by treatment of the adverse event, whether subjective symptoms or objective signs with a precisely verifiable onset are involved, and whether the latter are compatible with the natural history of the disease being treated; a grading system has been proposed (5). In any case, reviewing reported associations with a refined comprehension of the pharmacology of the drug, the disease under study, and relevant patient populations, may facilitate the identification of associations (6).

One of the first steps in the review of case reports is to focus on designated medical events (DMEs), e.g. adverse events which are rare, serious, and have a high drug-attributable risk distributed over multiple distinct pharmacological/therapeutic classes. It has been suggested that one to three reports may be considered a potential signal with these types of events. Typical examples include *aplastic anaemia, toxic epidermal necrolysis, Stevens-Johnson syndrome, Torsade de pointes, and hepatic failure, etc.* However, the definition is not absolute and there are some events that are considered DMEs even if they do not meet every one of the above criteria. An example is pancreatitis, for which the bulk of the risk is associated with alcohol use and gall bladder disease in adults. Furthermore, any event or set of events of special interest to an organization for specific surveillance or research purposes may be specified, and nothing prohibits them from attaching to these events the label "designated medical events" (7).

Naturally, there is no universally accepted or "correct" list of events of special interest, and variations on the concept exist. For example, the WHO Uppsala Monitoring Centre has a "critical terms" list of events that is indicative of serious disease states, pointing to the need for more decisive action. The United States FDA has a list of "Interesting PTs" (8). The EMA has a list that closely follows the list of serious events in CIOMS Working Group V (9). Other organizations customize their own lists.

Other events of specific interest, also referred to as targeted medical events (TMEs), are associated with particular medicinal products and/or patient populations. Operationally, they are treated in a similar manner to DMEs, but classification is drug-dependent. In this case, pharmacovigilance logic and a scientific knowledge of the drug, treatment indication, and/or relevant patient populations, allow prediction of potential issues that might emerge. These could be legitimate issues or issues that are, in effect, spurious from a causal perspective, but likely to be raised given the disease under study, the patient populations, and the potential biases and reporting artefacts inherent in SRS systems.

Other clinical features may evoke special attention. For example, hyperacute (so-called "end-of-the-needle") events usually require careful evaluation. These events involve a biologically plausible AE that occurs in extremely close temporal association to parenteral administration in otherwise stable circumstances. The clinical characteristics of the event itself may be sufficiently specific to infer at least a contributory role for the drug, e.g. a renal or biliary calculus composed of pure drug. Such events represent another type of report that may have high informational content (*10, 11*).

It is important to note that even beyond the DME and TME classification, the traditional methods of signal detection are not the automatic and mindless assessment of every reported association as a potential signal. There are other criteria that may be incorporated as part of the clinical triage of cases for the purposes of signal detection. For example, if a hypothetical drug is known to produce moderate respiratory depression and reports are submitted of apnoea/respiratory arrest, which would be considered unlabelled by virtue of severity the safety reviewer may well consider the established, but milder, form of the event, as biological justification to examine the newly reported, more severe event. Venulet has described the related concept of "discerning parameters" (*12*).

Generation and analysis of periodic reviews of safety of newly licensed products is viewed as another very important traditional signal detection tool in pharmacovigilance (*13*). Examples of such periodic aggregate reports include periodic safety update reports (PSURs) and annual safety reports (ASRs) in Europe, periodic adverse drug experience reports (PADERs) and IND safety reports in the United States, and J-PSURs in Japan. These reports, by virtue of line listings, summary tabulations and discussion of individual safety topics provide a comprehensive look at the data at a defined time point. Periodic reporting of aggregate data, e.g. in a PSUR, is often used by regulators and pharmaceutical companies as a tool for the ongoing review of pharmacovigilance and other information with a potential bearing on the benefit-risk balance and product labelling. The standard data included in such reports are amenable to this type of review, as they contain information on estimated usage, results from clinical studies, and experience in special populations, as well as descriptions of new and ongoing signal monitoring. In addition, safety reviews are conducted based on cumulative information from one review period to the next. In the EU there is also a link between the periodic reporting and the EU Risk Management Plans introduced at the end of 2005.

b. Simple analyses of larger datasets

Line listings and cumulative overview tables or both can be reviewed to identify unexpectedly high numbers of the same or similar AE reports. A signal is detected when a higher than expected value is observed for an adverse event or a group of adverse events in any of the following:

- Number of specific AE reports (absolute number);
- Number of specific AE reports / total number of reports for drug (proportion); or
- Number of specific AE reports / estimated exposure to drug (proportion).

In addition to providing a snapshot at a given time-point, such figures may be used to illustrate trends that are observed over the lifecycle of a product.

Of course, traditional methods implicitly or explicitly involve notions of the number of reports to be expected for a drug-event combination. The same applies to any rate or estimate derived from such a number. As with the more complex methods described later in this report, while a useful conceptual prop, it understandably is not possible to say what is truly "expected" with SRS data, given the numerous limitations mentioned above. It is important to note that a high prevalence within a case series of various case-specific features discussed above, under the individual striking case method, may also be one criterion that may potentially elevate the case series to signal status.

The methods of analysis of pharmacovigilance information have been reviewed previously. For example, the ICH E2E Guideline "Pharmacovigilance Planning" (*4 in Chapter I*) contains a high-level overview of the commonly accepted methods (see Table 4) (*14*). This ICH Guideline addresses the methods used in the conduct of pharmacovigilance on medicinal products during the post-authorisation phase across the life-cycle of a medicinal product. Other methods used during the pre-authorisation phase, mostly clinical trials and other systematic data collection schemes, have been subject to extensive review and have been described, for example, in the CIOMS Working Group VI report on the management of safety information from clinical trials (*15*).

Table 4: Post-authorisation pharmacovigilance methods[a] described in the ICH E2E Guideline

Data collection method	Examples
I. Passive surveillance	Spontaneous reports Case series
II. Stimulated reporting	Early Post-marketing Phase Vigilance (EPPV), Japan
III. Active surveillance	Sentinel sites Drug event monitoring / Prescription Event Monitoring (PEM), Registries
IV. Comparative observational studies	Cross-sectional study (survey) Case-control study Cohort study
V. Targeted clinical investigations	Genetic testing Special population trial Large simple trial
VI. Descriptive studies	Natural history of disease Drug utilisation study

[a] The methods listed represent examples and are not limited to initial signal detection.

The choice of methods for statistical signal detection depends on the type of data to be analysed, which, in turn, will depend on the method of data collection. Conceptually, in pharmacovigilance, as in public health in general, there are two major approaches – passive and active. In the first instance (passive surveillance), information about events of interest is submitted voluntarily/spontaneously by patients, or their healthcare providers, directly to the regulatory authorities or, indirectly, via manufacturers or distributors. In the second type of approach (active surveillance), information about events potentially associated with exposure to drugs is gathered proactively by pharmacovigilance practitioners via a specially designed schema/

survey (e.g. Prescription Event Monitoring) or from available electronic sources of patient data, e.g. administrative databases (see Table 5).

Table 5: Methods of data collection and signal detection in pharmacovigilance

Methods of PhV data collection	Methods of signal detection
Passive surveillance	
Routine collection of spontaneous reports (e.g. MedWatch or Vaccine Adverse Event Reporting System (VAERS) systems in the USA, Yellow Card system in the UK, EudraVigilance in the EEA) Targeted collection and extensive follow-up of certain report types (exposure/drug based, or outcome based), e.g. Varicella Vaccine Pregnancy Registry, CDC smallpox vaccination program (*16*), Biosurveillance programs (*17*)	Review of Designated Medical Events, or Targeted Medical Events[a] Review of other event reports for "striking" features (e.g. positive re-challenge)[a] Periodic aggregate review of spontaneous reports[a] Automated screening of adverse event databases, or data mining, for patterns of disproportionate reporting using reporting rate ratios
Active Surveillance	
Collection of product safety information via prescriber (as in Prescription Event Monitoring (*18*)) or patient surveys (e.g. Lareb Intensive Monitoring web-based program in Holland (*19*), or Immunization Monitoring Program ACTive (IMPACT) system in Canada) Via access to large linked databases containing claims data or electronic patient records	maxSPRT[b] method (for limited list of medical events) Screening analyses for elevated relative risks of a wide range of events, e.g. ICD9 diagnoses, in treated patients versus controls, or other similar statistics (e.g. information component)

[a] Items in a), b), and c) are referred to as traditional, manual, or conventional methods.
[b] maxSPRT – maximized Sequential Probability Ratio Testing (*20*, *21*).

c. Conclusions and recommendations

- Although SRS databases as a whole have numerous quality limitations and deficits, individual spontaneous reports and case series may have high clinical information value for the detection of signals.

- Traditional methods (case report and case series review, simple quantitative filters) are, and in the foreseeable future will continue to be, a foundation of signal detection activities using spontaneous reports.

- Effective screening and evaluation of individual reports and series of cases requires expert scientific judgement and experience. It is important that the value of multi-disciplinary expertise is not obscured by the focus on more sophisticated automated techniques.

- A strength of the periodic reports method, mandated by regulatory agencies, is the ability to routinely review aggregate data using simple quantitative parameters. Periodic review will continue to be required and used as an important signal detection tool. However, it is likely to be used in a more proportionate way focusing on the earlier part of a product life-cycle where knowledge of safety is accruing.

References

1. Amery WK. Signal generation from spontaneous adverse event reports. *Pharmacoepidemiology and Drug Safety*, 1999, 8(2):147-50.

2. Clark JA, Klincewicz SL, Stang PE. Spontaneous adverse event signalling methods: classification and use with health care treatment products. *Epidemiologic Review*, 2001, 23(2):191.

3. Clark JA, Klincewicz SL, Stang PE. Overview – spontaneous signalling. *Pharmacovigilance*, Mann RD, Andrews EB (eds) 247-271.

4. Begaud B et al. False positives in spontaneous reporting: should we worry about them? *British Journal of Clinical Pharmacology*, 1994, 38(5):401-4.

5. Girard M. Conclusiveness of re-challenge in the interpretation of adverse drug reactions 1987. *British Journal of Clinical Pharmacology*, 1987, 23:73-79.

6. Hauben M, Horn S, Reich L. Potential utility of data mining algorithms for the detection of "surprise" adverse drug reactions. *Drug Safety*, 2007, 30(2):143-155.

7. Hochberg AM, Hauben M. Time-to-signal comparison for drug safety data-mining algorithms vs. traditional signalling criteria. *Clinical Pharmacology & Therapeutics*, 2009, 85(6):600-606.

8. Bright RA, Nelson RC. Automated support for pharmacovigilance: a proposed system. *Pharmacoepidemiology and Drug Safety*, 2002, 11(2):121-5.

9. Report of CIOMS Working Group V. *Current challenges in pharmacovigilance: pragmatic approaches*. Geneva, CIOMS, 2001.

10. Aronson JK, Hauben M. Anecdotes that provide definitive evidence. *British Medical Journal*, 2006, 333:1267-1269.

11. Hauben M, Aronson JK. Gold standards in pharmacovigilance: the use of definitive anecdotal reports of adverse drug reactions as pure gold and high grade ore. *Drug Safety*, 2007, 30(8):645-55.

12. Venulet J. Possible strategies for early recognition of potential drug safety problems. *Adv. Drug React. Ac. Pois. Rev*, 1988, 1:39-47.

13. Klepper MJ. The periodic safety report as a pharmacovigilance tool. *Drug Safety*, 2004, 27(8):569-78.

14. ICH E2E *Guideline: Pharmacovigilance Planning*. 2004. (http://www.ich.org/LOB/media/MEDIA1195.pdf, accessed 19 August 2007).

15. *Management of safety information from clinical trials*. Report of CIOMS Working Group VI. Geneva, CIOMS, 2005. ISBN 92 9036 079 8.

16. Baggs J et al. Safety profile of smallpox vaccine: Insights from the laboratory worker smallpox vaccination program. *Clinical Infectious Diseases*, 2005, 40(8):1133-1140.

17. Hoffman MA et al. Multijurisdictional approach to biosurveillance, Kansas City. *Emerg Infect Dis*, 2003, 9(10):1281-1286. (http://www.cdc.gov/ncidod/EID/vol9no10/03-0060.htm, accessed 27 December 2007).

18. Ferreira G. Prescription-event monitoring: developments in signal detection. *Drug Safety*, 2007, 30(7):639-641.

19. Description of Lareb intensive monitoring system. (http://www.lareb.nl/kennis/monitor.asp, Dutch and English language sections accessed 19 August 2007).

20. Davis RL et al. Active surveillance of vaccine safety: a system to detect early signs of adverse events. *Epidemiology.* 2005 May, 16(3):336-41.

21. Brown JS et al. Early detection of adverse drug events within population-based health networks: application of sequential testing methods. *Pharmacoepidemiology and Drug Safety*, 2007, October 22. [Epub ahead of print] PMID: 17955500.

VII

More complex quantitative signal detection methods

a. History

Since the late 1990s there has been an intensified interest in the application of more complex methods to signal detection in pharmacovigilance. Most of these methods rely on comparisons of relative reporting frequencies, also known as disproportionality analyses; all of these methods incorporate several assumptions relating to the number of reports one would "expect" to be recorded in the database:

- When a specific medicinal product induces a specific adverse reaction, this reaction is reported more often for this medicine than with the other medicinal products that do not induce the AE, so that the magnitude of a disproportionality metric is likely to be increased;

- For the same reaction, the extent of (under)reporting is assumed to be the same amongst different medicinal products;

- The reporting rate of the reactions or the overall pattern of reporting is assumed to be a valid reference against which to compare the reporting of individual drug-event combinations.

These assumptions are weak in the sense that many counter-examples can be found, e.g. stimulated reporting/reporting artifacts.

Enhanced quantitative methods refer to computer-aided statistical methodologies and Data Mining Algorithms (DMAs) that, at the present time, mostly rely on disproportionality analysis (DA) based on 2x2 contingency tables (see Table 7) (*1*). These more recently developed methods are not designed to replace the traditional approaches, but are considered for their potential as a support tool for analyzing large volumes of data in a structured and auditable way. For many of the stakeholders in pharmacovigilance, these quantitative methods are seen as exploratory and not yet fully established in the pharmacovigilance systems. Table 6 describes some of the key historical landmarks in the evolution of this methodology in pharmacovigilance.

b. Disproportionality analysis – general concepts and caveats

The basic objective of disproportionality analysis (DA) is to identify statistically prominent reporting associations between pairs of drugs and events within SRS databases. What is considered statistically prominent is determined by what might be expected by chance, which is related to the proportionate representation of drugs (across all events) and events (across all or most drugs). The finding of a statistic of disproportionate reporting (SDR) (the term used for the numerical outputs of these analyses devoid of clinical context) does not mean that a signal of suspected causality exists (*20, 21*). The following aspects should be taken into account when considering observed SDRs.

Table 6: A history of quantitative methods in pharmacovigilance

Year method published	Comment
1968	Napke designed a cabinet he called the "pigeon hole" for the Health Canada SRS. One dimension of the cabinet defined drugs and other adverse events. Each drug-event combination had a separate hole or slot. Coloured tabs were attached to reports of severe or unusual AEs allowing the visual detection of drug-event combinations. Although not a computer-assisted system, the "pigeon-hole" approach represented an innovative way to visualize SRS data (*2*).
1969	Patwary suggested the use of 2x2 contingency tables to monitor for changes in drug-specific reporting frequency over time. This became known as "Patwary signalling" (*3*).
1973	Venulet reported a routine implementation of signalling on the WHO drug safety monitoring center database using a computer system. The method was described as follows: "When the level of reporting to a drug expressed as a ratio between the number of reports concerning this drug and the total number of reports for a given time period, or batch of reports differs from a preceding ratio calculated for another period of time or batch of reports, a signal is generated by the computer" (*4*).
1974	Finney, in a review of automated signalling in SRS databases, proposed several new approaches/methods. One of them, termed Reaction Proportion Signalling, became later known as PRR (Proportionate Reporting Ratio) screening. Finney defined the method as follows: "[The method] involves comparison of records for a single drug and reaction, with those for a larger set of drugs and reactions. ... Note that the frequencies should be counts of cases or reports, not of drug-reaction combinations" (*5*).
1976	Mandel et al., proposed novel methods for looking for sudden increases in reporting in SRS data, and the methods were extended further by Levine et al. in 1977 (*6, 7*).
1992	The first peer-reviewed publication by Stricker and Tijssen applying Reporting Odds Ratio methodology to a WHO Monitoring Centre's database to evaluate a drug safety issue was published in the Journal of Clinical Epidemiology (*8*).
1996	The first publication describing a method of comparing relative events proportions (termed "proportional morbidity distributions") for two different vaccine products in the Vaccine Adverse Events Reporting System is presented by vaccine safety researchers (Rosenthal et al) at the Centers for Disease Control and Prevention (CDC) (*9*).
1997	Disproportionality analysis used in a publication by Moore et al investigating the reporting association between hypoglycemia and ACE inhibitors. First use of the term "case-not-case" to describe the methodology, first suggested by Begaud in 1983 (*10*).
1998	World Health Organization Uppsala Monitoring Centre (Bate et al) pioneered the application of Bayesian methodology to 2x2 contingency tables (Bayesian Confidence Propagation Neural Network or BCPNN) for signal detection in SRS data bases (*11*).

Year method published	Comment
1998	Evans "rediscovered" Finney's Reaction Proportion Signalling and coins the term "Proportional Reporting Ratio". PRR became a signal detection method routinely used on the UK national spontaneous reports database.
1999	A variation of the above Bayesian methodology for 2x2 tables, the Multi-item Gamma-Poisson shrinker (MGPS) introduced by DuMouchel (*12*).
2001	Exploration of Bayesian disproportionality analysis for pattern recognition of drug-associated syndromes presented by WHO (*13*).
2002	Purcell (TGA) and Barty developed 'PROFILE,' an iterative probability filtering algorithm based on Fisher's Exact Test, to take 'innocent bystander' drugs into consideration (*14*).
2003	Researchers at the CDC demonstrated how a large electronic health/medical records database could be used to screen for a number of non *a priori* suspected outcomes of interest following vaccination using a conventional cohort analysis approach (i.e. screening for disproportionate Risk Ratios) (Verstraeten et al). This represented the earliest published example of active surveillance and data mining in longitudinal patient records databases (*15*).
2003	Joint PhRMA-FDA Safety Evaluation Tools (SET) Working Group formed.
2004-5	Bate published on Information Component difference mining in IMS (the UK) database – the first attempt to apply active surveillance to drugs using a data mining method originally developed for SRS databases on a longitudinal patient records database (*16*).
2005	European Medicines Evaluation Agency (EMEA) EudraVigilance Expert Working Group signal detection subgroup formed.
2005	USA FDA issued *Guidance for Industry Good Pharmacovigilance Practices and Pharmaco-epidemiological Assessment* that contains a section discussing quantitative methods (*17*).
2005	PhRMA-FDA SET Working group published a white paper on data mining in pharmacovigilance.
2006	CIOMS Working Group VIII on Practical Aspects of Signal Detection in Pharmacovigilance was formed.
2007	EMEA released guidance to specifically address in detail the use of quantitative approaches in pharmacovigilance: *Guideline on the Use of Statistical Signal Detection Methods in the EudraVigilance Data Analysis System*, Doc. Ref. EMEA/106464/2006 rev.1 (*18*).
2009	MHRA published Good Vigilance Practice Guide (*19*).

A statistical reporting relationship does not necessarily imply a causal relationship. It may reflect one or more of a number of biases and artefacts inherent in pharmacovigilance data as well as "statistical noise". Consequently, there is a scientific consensus that SDRs identified with quantitative methods should always be viewed through the lens of scientific knowledge, judgement and experience prior to concluding that not just an SDR but a signal of suspected causality exists that warrants a complete medical evaluation (*22*). This is in keeping with the description of "signal" by Meyboom et al. that a signal consists of both data and arguments (*23*).

Statistical analysis of SRS data entails subjective decisions in the selection, deployment and interpretation of data mining procedures and outputs and accordingly, results may not be generalizable (*24*). The initial decision on whether a drug-event combination is numerically distinctive in these models is obviously based in part on the numerical thresholds selected. Currently, there is no "gold standard" for determining which threshold(s) should be adopted to define an SDR although several metric/threshold combinations are commonly used or endorsed (*25*). The thresholds commonly used to detect SDRs are a trade-off between two options: either generating too many 'false positive signals' if the threshold is too low or missing 'potential signals' if this threshold is too high.

The value of disproportionality statistics depends significantly on the database from which the measures of disproportionality are computed. Initial interpretation of disproportionality calculations should therefore take relevant elements into account, such as:

- The type of medicinal products (and indications for use) included in the database;

- The medical terminology(ies) applied, including consideration of data that has been migrated from one terminology to another over time, and individual term selection and coding practices (particularly coding conventions and dictionary versioning) (*26*);

- The date of the creation of the database;

- The reporting source(s) and collection methods of ICSRs, i.e. all unsolicited reports; and

- The origin of the ICSRs (national, regional, other country) since the indications or dosing for the same medicinal product may vary across countries and regions.

These and other elements can influence the number and magnitude of the SDRs and/or their interpretation and may introduce various biases or distortions such as masking effects, in which a distinctive reporting association is obscured by a strong reporting association of that event with another drug(s). Alternatively, they may exaggerate the magnitude of a medicinal product-adverse event statistical association that may or may not reflect causality. The absence of an SDR does not necessarily exclude the possibility of a causal association between the medicinal product and the adverse event.

Caution should be exercised when comparing disproportionality calculations between more than one medicinal product. Such comparisons may not lead to reliable conclusions due to the biases involved, e.g. stages of the products' life cycles, stimulated reporting, differences in overall safety profiles, etc. In this circumstance, it is possible that biases and reporting artefacts may add or multiply together. Results from disproportionality analysis, including results for individual drugs and comparisons between drugs, may be especially difficult to interpret when spontaneous reporting is unstable or in disequilibrium, as when an association is the subject of publicity or media attention with resulting stimulated reporting (*27, 28*).

Measures of disproportionate reporting calculated from SRS data merely provide another perspective on reporting behaviour at a point in time. They cannot be used to explain the cause of quantitatively distinctive reporting behaviour, which may reflect causality, but could also reflect chance, recorded or unrecorded confounding factors and/or various reporting artefacts. In other words, an SDR in and of itself neither proves nor implies causality. This cannot be overemphasised, especially as techniques with an extensive mathematical approach may seduce users into minimizing or forgetting the fundamental quantitative and qualitative defects in some of the datasets used for signal detection, most notably in SRS data. It also emphasizes that statistical calculations on SRS data should not be viewed in a biological vacuum (29).

c. Theory of disproportionality analysis

(1) Basic methodologies and metrics

As discussed in detail below, the most commonly used methods of disproportionality analysis may be classified according to whether they are based on a classical or frequentist statistical paradigm (i.e. probabilities viewed as a long term frequency with an assumption of a repeatable experiment or sampling mechanism) or a Bayesian paradigm (probability as a degree of belief that formally incorporates prior beliefs or knowledge that is updated in light of new information). However, the fundamental calculations are more similar than different and the basic theory described below in this section is applicable to both approaches.

The common feature of DMAs that support disproportionality analysis is that they condense very complex safety datasets onto 2x2 contingency tables for each drug-event combination. The statistical 2x2 table has commonly been used in drug safety and is the basis for various calculations of association measures. This 2x2 table may be viewed as a "book-keeping" device that tallies the number of reports according to the presence or absence of drug and events of interest, as shown in Table 7.

Table 7: Contingency table used in disproportionality analysis

	Reports for event of interest	Reports for all other events	Total
Reports for drug of interest	A	B	A+B
Reports for all other drugs	C	D	C+D
Total	**A+C**	**B+D**	**A+B+C+D**

Certain patterns may be noted in such a table according to whether and to what degree a given drug and event of interest are associated. For example, if the drug and event are positively associated they may tend to be reported together or not appear together quite often in the database with higher counts in cells A and D. If they are negatively associated, then the drug may often appear without the event and vice versa, which may favour reports falling into cells B and C.

Various statistical measures of association may be calculated from a contingency table that reflect the strength of the association, such as reporting odds ratios (RORs), relative reporting (RR) and proportional reporting ratio (PRR). For each such metric a range of values in the form of a confidence interval is often calculated based on the frequentist statistical notion of repeated sampling. The two most commonly used frequentist methods are PRRs and RORs. Commonly used association metrics are listed in Table 8. Use of the lower limit of such intervals as a threshold in signal detection is one mechanism for mitigating false positive findings, which is especially pertinent to associations with low observed and/or expected counts. Another approach is the use of a multiplicity correction (*30*).

Table 8: Common measures of association for 2x2 tables used in disproportionality analysis

Measure of Association	Formula	Probabilistic Interpretation
Relative reporting (RR) (*31*)	$\dfrac{A(A + B + C + D)}{(A + C)(A + B)}$	$\dfrac{Pr(ae \mid drug)}{Pr(ae)}$
Proportional reporting ratio (PRR)	$\dfrac{A(C + D)}{C(A + B)}$	$\dfrac{Pr(ae \mid drug)}{Pr(ae \mid {\sim} drug)}$
Reporting odds ratio (ROR)	$\dfrac{AD}{CB}$	$\dfrac{Pr(ae \mid drug)\, Pr({\sim} ae \mid {\sim} drug)}{Pr({\sim} ae \mid drug)\, Pr(ae \mid {\sim} drug)}$
Information component (IC)	$Log_2 \dfrac{A(A + B + C + D)}{(A + C)(A + D)}$	$\dfrac{Log_2\, Pr(ae \mid drug)}{Pr(ae)}$

The literature contains comparisons of the various association metrics (*32*), but detailed debates on, for example, the relative merits of reporting odds ratios versus proportional reporting ratios are rare (*33, 34, 35*). There is much more debate on the advantages and disadvantages of calculating the values of the above association metrics within a frequentist versus a Bayesian framework (discussed further below in section 3) that ultimately reduce to consideration of the sensitivity, specificity and predictive value of each approach.

A fundamental principle applicable to any signal detection method is that focusing exclusively on minimizing false positives may preclude useful knowledge discovery, while focusing exclusively on reducing false negatives may be self-defeating by flooding the system with an overabundance of signals that divert valuable resources. Quantifying these trade-offs remains a challenge (*36*).

After almost a decade of development, testing, and implementation of data mining in pharmacovigilance, this approach has reportedly enhanced signal detection practices at some major pharmacovigilance organizations, but results are variable. Some organizations, such as the WHO Uppsala Monitoring Centre, which does not have access to case narratives and relies heavily on numerical summaries, may be uniquely positioned to benefit from data mining, but any organization responsible for screening large repositories of spontaneous reports may consider data mining a credible option for enhancing signal detection activities. On the other hand, in many organizations, data mining has identified associations that are already known, under evaluation, or deemed non-causal after evaluation. It is important to note that an observation that a

DMA highlights many already known causal associations, may, but does not necessarily, indicate lack of utility for that organization. In some sense it is reassuring that known associations are being highlighted, akin to positive controls, and more information would be needed before a conclusion could be reached about incremental value or signal detection performance, e.g. does the DMA highlight the known associations before, concurrently, or after, traditional signalling protocols, and with how much person-time expended. Taken together, the cumulative knowledge and experience to date suggests that a realistic view would fall somewhere between the extremes of "unbridled optimism" and "considerable pessimism" noted by Bate and Edwards and that both the strengths and weakness of these methods should be carefully considered (37).

Example of a frequentist approach

Figure 2 is a temporal plot derived from a DMA, the proportional reporting ratio (PRR). The plot over time is a graphical output developed by Evans (38) depicting the evolution of a PRR for a given drug-event combination as data accumulates over time. This illustrates how a DMA can offer more than just numerical calculations and may include graphical and data visualization functionalities that can facilitate signal detection.

Figure 2. Temporal plot of PRRs for Isotretinoin and reports of depression

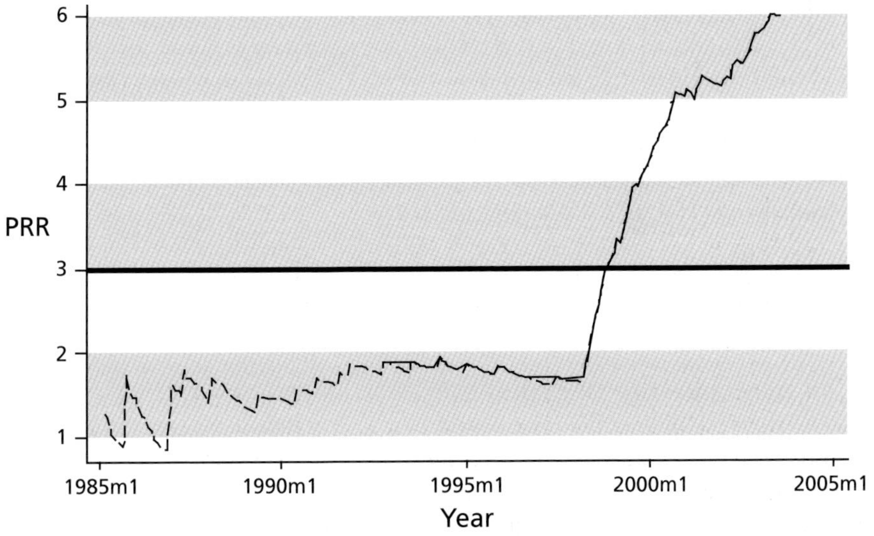

(2) Bayesian methodologies

While analysis of disproportionate reporting in pharmacovigilance is not a recent invention (39), two aspects associated with this methodology have resulted in a renewed interest in this type of tool. First is the technological capacity for rapidly calculating measures of association on millions of 2x2 tables. In a database that contains in the order of 15,000 drug names and 16,000 adverse event preferred terms, there may be approximately 240 million corresponding 2x2 tables, one for each drug-event combination. Enumeration of all possible tables and corresponding association metrics is tedious, but still within existing hardware capabilities (40).

The application of Bayesian statistical approaches to signal detection in pharmacovigilance, pioneered by the World Health Organization Uppsala Monitoring Centre in the late 1990s, has resulted in renewed interest in disproportionality analysis. The two major Bayesian methods in use are the Bayesian Confidence Propagation Neural Network (BCPNN) and the Multi-item Gamma Poisson Shrinker (MGPS). The existence of large, sparse databases, a focus on rare events in pharmacovigilance, and the use of hypergranular adverse events dictionaries, means that safety reviewers are frequently confronted with drug-event combinations whose 2x2 tables often have a low number of observed and/or expected reports in cell A, i.e. the cell containing the number of instances in which both the drug of interest and the event of interest are listed in the same report. The great majority of theoretically possible drug-event combinations in large regulatory databases, for example, will have very few or even no such combinations actually reported.

In the absence of prior knowledge or biological plausibility, an observed/ expected (O/E) ratio based on five cases may be less indicative of demonstrably disproportionate reporting (increased O/E) than one based on 50 cases. In the former instance, the calculated association metrics may have large calculated variances, with many elevated (low) O/E ratios generated by low numbers of reports, decreasing (increasing) to greater or lesser degrees with the accumulation of additional reports. With asymptotic assumptions, which may not necessarily be appropriate in this context, this can be expressed as a standard error for the various association metrics, which, in this setting, will be dominated by a low number of reports in cell A (reports of the drug-event of interest). Frequentist methods have typically addressed this challenge using statistical significance/unexpectedness thresholds and/or confidence intervals. Recently, frequentist multiplicity corrections have also been applied to mitigate the variance challenge in sparse databases (*see 30*).

While frequentist approaches address the variability associated with low numbers of reports by calculation of confidence intervals and the use of multiplicity corrections, the Bayesian methods attempt to address highly variable O/Es with low observed or expected reporting frequencies by first calculating an association metric that is similar to PRR (RR in Table 8) but in a rough sense averaged over the entire database, or set equal to one. This serves as a null RR or O/E value for all drug-event combinations (DECs) that is subsequently combined via a statistical weighting scheme based on Bayes' rule with the value of the associated metric that is calculated for the individual DEC/2x2 table. Thus the calculated association O/E metric is a composite value that will fall somewhere between the overall average or null value and the value based on the 2x2 table for the individual DEC. When there are no reports or the number of observed or expected reports is low, the weighted composite will equal or fall much closer to the null value. Larger values for the individual DEC based on small numbers of reports that might possibly represent chance fluctuations are thus reduced towards the null value. This is the so-called Bayesian "shrinkage" of the "crude" O/E when the observed and/or expected counts are low. "Shrinkage" is when the initially calculated O/E that exceeds the null value is pulled or decreased to or towards one or the null value, the value we would expect if drug and event were independent of each other in the database (note that O/Es that are less than the null value may be "pulled up" or increased towards the null value). This is a reasonable approach in terms of minimizing overall error, but may be erroneous for some DECs. Each Bayesian method accomplishes the above in fundamentally the same way, although specific implementation details vary.

Another rough conceptualization is that the Bayesian methods make a first guess or embody an underlying assumption that, due to sampling variability in a 'noisy' post-marketing database, the true O/Es of most associations are closer together and closer to one than they would appear to be, based on the observed "sample" database. It should be stressed that the notion that the SRS database is a sample from an infinite ensemble of spontaneous reports may be useful for explanatory purposes, but may not be accurate and may inappropriately frame signal detection as an estimation procedure rather than exploratory and descriptive data analysis.

The overall reporting experience, or pattern of reporting frequencies of all drug-event combinations (DECs), is the source of not just the overall mean O/E but the so-called prior probability distributional assumption of O/Es yielding the overall O/E of one or close to one, as well as an associated spread or range of plausible O/E ratios around that overall mean. Therefore, Bayesian methods simultaneously accommodate and assess multiple possible O/Es or hypotheses from the start, in addition to the overall null O/E value. How narrow or wide the spread of the prior distribution is will determine the degree of shrinkage towards the null. All else being equal, a narrow prior distribution that is very concentrated around the null value, akin to the effect of a larger sample size, will be associated with more intense shrinkage towards the null value than a prior distribution that is more diffusely spread about the null value, akin to a smaller sample size. Because the first guess actually includes a point "estimate" and a range of plausible values, some researchers contend that such terminology (e.g. "estimate") implies an inappropriate equation of exploratory data analysis with epidemiological estimation (41).

For each specific DEC, this prior probability is then adjusted or updated, via Bayes' rule, to produce an updated mean and range of possible O/Es and associated probabilities for that specific DEC. This distribution of updated O/Es is the so-called posterior probability distribution. To recap, the posterior distribution reflects something of a weighted average of the overall grand mean O/E and the O/E ratio for the specific DEC of interest. Although the prior information may in a sense be biased, it is based on a very large corpus of data and considered to have low variability, i.e. stable to small changes in the numbers of reports. Therefore, it is weighted quite heavily at first until the number of reports of the specific DEC of interest achieves a critical mass, at which point its influence dominates the weighted average. This may be viewed as building in an element of initial scepticism under limited information. The major difference between BCPNN and MGPS is that they fit different families of distributions to construct the prior probability distributions and do the data fitting in different ways.

The "shrinkage" metrics, which again are Bayesian implementations of the simple metrics listed in Table 8, are known by a variety of names, including the information component (IC) in the BCPNN and the Empirical Bayes Geometric Mean

(EBGM) in MGPS. Each of these metrics has an associated credibility interval with commonly used upper and lower cut-points, i.e. the lower fifth percentile of the empirical Bayes gamma mixture (EB05). Note that the initialism "EBGM" has been used to refer to two distinct concepts in the published literature: the Empirical Bayes Gamma Mixture, as well as the Empirical Bayes Geometric Mean.

Example of the Bayesian approach

Figure 3 is a time scan generated by a DMA, the Bayesian confidence propagation neural network (BCPNN). The time scan is a graphical output developed by the WHO Uppsala Monitoring Centre that depicts the temporal evolution of the O/E for a given DEC as data accumulates over time. This illustrates how contemporary DMAs offer more than just numerical calculations, and not only may include numerous graphical and data visualization functionalities that can facilitate signal detection, but also allow for case level drill-down of the data. In addition to enabling familiarization with graphical data mining outputs and capabilities, Figure 3 provides an informative data display to demonstrate the underlying dynamic process involved in disproportionality analysis of any sort over time.

Figure 3. Time scan of Suprofen and reports of back pain

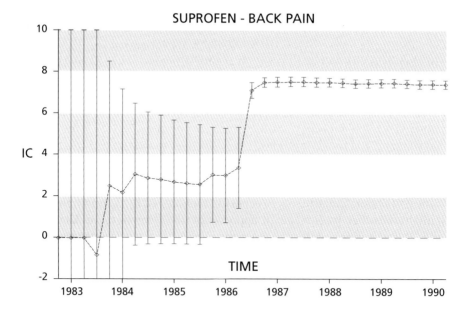

It is instructive to examine the evolution of this SDR over time as different reports, e.g. with and without the drug or event of interest, are entered into the database to reinforce understanding the underlying process of disproportionality analysis. The IC is initially zero, meaning that the O/E is 1 ($\log_2 1 = 0$). This reflects the prior assumption of independence between the drug and the event. This physically corresponds to the absence of reports for the target drug so that the shrinkage or null value O/E of 1 applies. The confidence intervals (CIs) are wide due to the limited data. Beginning in mid-1983, the IC becomes negative (O/E < 1, log2 (O/E < 0) and the CIs begin to narrow. This corresponds to the fact that reports involving suprofen and other events are being entered in the database. The additional reports involving suprofen and other events, along with back pain reported for other drugs, increases the expected count of this combination without a concomitant increase in the observed count. Then, beginning in the last quarter of 1983, the IC becomes positive with the first report of the combination because the expected count is low (at this point there were only 46 reports in total with suprofen). Note that the credibility intervals initially remain wide in the setting of limited information, but the IC increases and the intervals narrow as additional reports of the combination accrue. By the 4th quarter of 1985 the third report of the combination results in the lower limit of the 95% CI exceeding zero, which could be considered an SDR.

(3) Frequentist versus Bayesian approaches

In practical terms, with low observed and/or expected cell counts, Bayesian methods applied to SRS data will tend to give lower relative reporting rate ratios than frequentist methods and will highlight fewer associations involving low cell counts at a given point in time because many will be "shrunk" towards independence (towards one), all else being equal. Of course whether and to what extent results from frequentist versus Bayesian methods differ depends on the specific implementation details of each method. Many of these associations may reflect spurious associations and Bayesian methods provide an elegant and effective approach to mitigating false positive findings that arise in the setting of limited information, but there may be trade-offs with respect to the risks of "shrinking" credible associations along with spurious associations. While overall accuracy has advantages, a data mining algorithm or protocol that allows a greater number of less serious errors to reduce the number of more serious errors may also have advantages. In the absence of a clear understanding of the frequency and consequences of classification errors in pharmacovigilance, it is difficult to declare one algorithm or class of algorithms or data mining protocol as providing *the* superior approach for all reported associations for all situations (*see 40*).

Similarly, associations that are eventually highlighted by both approaches may be highlighted earlier by frequentist approaches when common implementations are used, although minimum case count thresholds are used less frequently with Bayesian methods. This emphasizes the importance of considering not just what is or is not highlighted by one or another method at a given time point, but the importance of timeliness of signal detection (*42, 43*). Practically speaking, the performance of frequentist methods tends to converge with that of Bayesian methods when there are five or more reports of a drug-event pair, although larger gradients have been reported in specific scenarios (*see 32, 44, 45, 46, 47*).

(4) Evaluating data mining performance

Two questions about the more complex quantitative signal detection methods that may loom large in readers' minds is whether they are actually effective relative to traditional methods and whether there is a single or preferred method/approach (e.g.

frequentist versus Bayesian). These are not trivial questions and would require an extended exposition to fully flesh out the arguments but we discuss some key points.

As stated above, the more complex methods are established as credible additions to the pharmacovigilance tool kit that are reported to improve signal detection performance at some major pharmacovigilance organizations, but reported performance of these methods demonstrates substantial variation. Therefore, whether and to what degree they add incremental value to a given organization's signal detection activities may be highly situation dependent. Results may not only vary from organization to organization but may even vary from drug to drug. For example, the value of these approaches may be very different for new versus established drugs (48). Obviously, the incremental value of any signal detection methodology will depend on its placement within an organization's pre-existing suite of signal detection strategies and methods. Therefore it is difficult to make generalizations by extrapolating from data mining exercises to real-world pharmacovigilance scenarios. It is important to point out, however, that most traditional pharmacovigilance methods have not been rigorously validated either, though there is a longer history with their use.

The majority of published validation exercises involve retrospective evaluations of authentic SRS data based on a screening paradigm, and many are referenced throughout this report. A smaller number of published validation exercises involve the use of simulated data sets (49, 50). Some use both authentic data and simulated data (51, 52).

These published validation exercises report highly variable performance, expressed as sensitivity, specificity, receiver operator characteristic (ROC) curves, predictive value and/or number needed to detect. Therefore, despite a fairly extensive literature on this issue it is still not clear to what extent data mining in general improves organizational signal detection performance relative to traditional approaches and whether the differences in statistical properties between data mining metrics and algorithms translate into real-world pharmacovigilance scenarios. Indeed, some researchers have pointed out that, outside the somewhat artificial environment of isolated data mining exercises, it would be very challenging to determine how and whether statistical properties between individual metrics/methods actually translate into clinically significant differences in performance (16 in Chapter IV).

The following are some of the issues that complicate the performance assessment and validation of data mining in pharmacovigilance:

- The construction of gold standard sets of reference adverse events (i.e. "true positives" and "true negatives") against which to test the performance of quantitative methods is a fundamental challenge for which there is not yet a consensus approach (53).

- Contemporary disproportionality analysis entails making arbitrary selections from a large number of available choices that essentially defines the configuration of a given data mining "run". This has two important corollaries. First, the abundance of analytical options maximizes exploratory capacity but also underscores published warnings against falling prey to confirmation bias by trying to retrospectively fit a data mining analysis to pre-existing expectations (*54*). Second, performance gradients between methods may relate to the intrinsic properties of the methods, the details of the specific implementation of each method in a given data mining exercise, or some combination of the above.

- Some analytical choices impact on performance by influencing the actual numerical outputs. Examples, beyond the fundamental selections of algorithm, metric and threshold, include:
  - ❏ Database e.g. public versus proprietary or internal (*55, 56, 57*)
  - ❏ Whether to mine using suspect drugs only versus suspect plus concomitant
  - ❏ Whether the entire database is used as a background for comparison or specific subsets of the database (*see 35*)
  - ❏ Whether the analysis attempts to control for confounding by basic covariate stratification (*58, 59, 60*)
  - ❏ Which level of the adverse event or drug dictionary hierarchy is mined (61, 62).

- Bayesian methods provide one elegant solution to the false positive burden associated with large sparse databases.

- Operational choices may impact on signal detection performance by determining the response to a given numerical output (e.g. whether the results are used in series or in parallel with traditional methods to declare a signal).

- Some factors are less easy to assess and rarely included in published data mining exercises. An example is the process by which an SDR is evaluated. An analyst may select for review only those reports listing the statistically highlighted PT or may select reports for review involving not only the statistically highlighted PTs but medically related PTs as well. Such procedural variations may result in different performance and performance gradients between methods (*see 36*). Another is computational intensity, which determines the time needed to complete a data mining analysis and may vary substantially between different algorithms. This does not necessarily affect the actual numerical outputs or the response to an SDR but can have practical implications for performance in real-world pharmacovigilance scenarios (*63*).

- Other factors, including the inherent mathematical properties of individual data mining algorithms, may contribute to variability in findings and thus complicate performance assessment (*see 24*).

- When comparing newer methods to traditional methods, retrospectively pinpointing when a signal first appeared on the "radar screen" via traditional methods, versus when it was finally adjudicated and an action was taken, may be challenging but failure to do so could introduce a bias into comparative assessments (*64*).

- Finally, there is no consensus on a theoretical calculus of costs and utilities associated with different ranges of sensitivity and specificity and different errors in classification (e.g. how many false positives findings are justified to detect a true drug-associated interstitial nephritis six months earlier?).

d. Disclosure and review of potential conflict of interest

One of the positive ancillary effects of the explosion of interest in applying data mining software to pharmacovigilance is the increased number of collaborative relationships between pharmaceutical companies, regulatory authorities, software vendors and other stakeholders. However, there is a concomitantly increased potential for conflicts of interest and/or the appearance of such, and it is important that all potential conflicts of interest be clearly disclosed in public presentations and publications on data mining in pharmacovigilance to the extent that is practically feasible. Commercial conflicts of interest and ethical issues in study design are perhaps the most widely recognized and discussed in biomedical sciences (*65*), but intellectual conflicts of interest may also occur. In addition to the above mentioned recommended disclosure policy, an awareness by readers of the full range of possible competing interests, both commercial and intellectual, may facilitate navigating the data mining literature. The following definition of conflict of interest from the biomedical literature may be a useful point of orientation in this regard: "A conflict of interest occurs when the pursuit of a secondary objective has an inappropriate influence over the attainment of a primary objective. In the context of a medical journal, primary objectives are to describe research accurately, and to discuss interpretations and limitations fairly. A secondary objective may be anything (financial gain, a personal relationship, intellectual passion) that leads an author to overstate or denigrate research results, selectively withhold pertinent data or discussion, or exaggerate or minimize the shortcomings of research" (*66*).

e. Conclusions and recommendations

- The pharmacovigilance toolkit has significantly expanded in the last decade to include additional credible quantitative 2x2 table-based methods of varying degrees of complexity, often referred to as data mining algorithms.

- Data mining has enhanced the signal detection performance at major pharmacovigilance organizations but results may be highly situation dependent.

- Pharmacovigilance organizations charged with screening large safety databases composed of spontaneous reports may be especially well positioned to enhance their effectiveness by supplementing, or possibly replacing, some traditional approaches with data mining analysis.

- Despite the aggressive promotion of some DMAs, claims of universal superiority of a given DMA or class of DMAs must be viewed with circumspection in light of the complexity and residual uncertainty in the evaluation of classifier performance.

- Each DMA or class of DMAs may have their unique advantages and disadvantages, and their statistical properties may not translate into clinically significant differences (*67*). Key local decisions relate to threshold setting and other issues which will be situation dependent.

References

1. Hauben M et al. The role of data mining in pharmacovigilance. *Expert Opinion on Drug Safety*, 2005, 4(5):929-948.

2. Napke E. Drug adverse reaction alerting program. *Canadian Pharmacists Journal 20* (1968) 251-254.

3. Patwary KW. *Reports on statistical aspects of the pilot research project for international drug monitoring*. Confidential report prepared for WHO, Geneva, 1969.

4. Venulet J. Adverse reactions to drugs. WHO research centre. *International Journal of Clinical Pharmacology*, 1973 Apr, 7(2):253-64.

5. Finney DJ. Systematic signalling of adverse reactions to drugs. *Methods Inf Med*. 1974 Jan, 13(1):1-10.

6. Mandel SP, Levine A, Beleno GE. Signalling increases in reporting in international monitoring of adverse reactions to therapeutic drugs. *Methods Inf Med*, 1976. 15(1):1-10.

7. Levine A, Mandel SP, Santamaria A. Pattern signalling in health information monitoring systems. *Methods Inf Med*, 1977, 16(3):138-44.

8. Stricker BH, Tijssen JG. Serum sickness-like reactions to cefaclor. *Journal of Clinical Epidemiology*, 1992 Oct, 45(10):1177-84.

9. Rosenthal S, Chen R, Hadler S. The safety of acellular pertussis vaccine vs whole-cell pertussis vaccine. A postmarketing assessment. *Archives of Pediatric & Adolescent Medicine*. 1996 May, 150(5):457-60.

10. Moore N et al. Reports of hypoglycemia associated with the use of ACE inhibitors and other drugs: a case/non-case study in the French pharmacovigilance system data base. *British Journal of Clinical Pharmacology*, 1997, 44:513-18.

11. Bate A et al. A Bayesian neural network method for adverse drug reaction signal generation. *European Journal of Clinical Pharmacology*, 1998 June, 54(4):315-21.

12. DuMouchel W. Bayesian data mining in large frequency tables, with an application to the FDA spontaneous reporting system. *American Statistics*, 1999 Aug, 53(8):177-190.

13. Bate A et al. *Pattern recognition using a recurrent neural network and its application to the WHO data base*. 17th International Conference on Pharmacoepidemiology, Toronto, Canada, 2001. Orre R et al. A Bayesian recurrent neural network for unsupervised pattern recognition in large incomplete data sets. *International Journal of Neural Systems*, 2005, 15: 207-222.

14. Purcell P, Barty S. Statistical techniques for signal generation: the Australian experience. *Drug Safety*, 2002, 25(6):415-421.

15. Verstraeten T et al.; Vaccine Safety Datalink Team. Safety of thimerosal-containing vaccines: a two-phased study of computerized health maintenance organization databases. *Pediatrics*. 2003 Nov, 112(5):1039-48.

16. Bate A. Bayesian confidence propagation neural network. *Drug Safety*, 2007, 30(7):623-625.

17. FDA *Guidance for Industry: good pharmacovigilance practices and pharmacoepidemiological assessment*.

18. EMEA *Guideline on the use of statistical signal detection methods in the EudraVigilance data analysis system*, Doc. Ref. EMEA/106464/2006 rev.1.

19. The MHRA *Good Pharmacovigilance Practice Guide*. 2009. The Pharmaceutical Press, ISBN 978 0 85369 834 0.

20. Hauben M, Reich L, Chung S. Postmarketing surveillance of potentially fatal reactions to oncology drugs: potential utility of two signal detection algorithms. *European Journal of Clinical Pharmacology*, 2004, 60(1):747-750.

21. Hauben M, Reich L. Communication of findings in pharmacovigilance: use of the term "signal" and the need for precision in its use. *European Journal of Clinical Pharmacology*, 2005, 61(5-5):479-480.

22. Hauben M, Aronson J. Defining 'signal' and its subtypes in pharmacovigilance based on a systematic review of previous definitions. *Drug Safety*, 2009, 32(2):99-110.

23. Meyboom RHB et al. Signal selection and follow-up in pharmacovigilance. *Drug Safety*, 2002, 25(6):459-465.

24. Hauben M et al. Illusions of objectivity and a recommendation for reporting data mining results. *European Journal* of *Clinical Pharmacology*, 2007; 63(5):517-21.

25. Szarfman A, Machado S, O'Neill RT. Use of screening algorithms and computer systems to efficiently signal combinations of drugs in the US FDA's spontaneous reports database. *Drug Safety*, 2002, 25(6):381-392.

26. Hauben M, Reich L. Valproate-induced Parkinsonism: use of a newer pharmacovigilance tool to investigate the reporting of an unanticipated adverse event with an "old" drug. *Movement Disorders*, 2005, 20(3): 387.

27. Moore N et al. Biases affecting the proportional reporting ratio (PPR) in spontaneous reports databases: the example of sertindole. *Pharmacoepidemiology and Drug Safety*, 2003, 12(4):271-281.

28. Pariente A et al. Effect of date of drug marketing on disproportionality measures in pharma-covigilance. The example of suicide with SSRIs using data from the UK MHRA. *Drug Safety*, 2009, 32(5):441-47.

29. Hauben M et al. Data mining in pharmacovigilance: the need for a balanced perspective. *Drug Safety*, 2005, 28(10):835-842.

30. Hochberg AM et al. Using data mining to predict safety actions from FDA adverse events reporting system data. *Drug Information Journal*, 2007, 41:633-43.

31. IC and RR formulated in a Bayesian framework in BCPNN and M(GPS), respectively.

32. van Puijenbroek EP et al. A comparison of measures of disproportionality for signal detection in spontaneous reporting systems for adverse drug reactions. *Pharmacoepidemiology and Drug Safety*, 2002, 11:3-10.

33. Rothman KJ, Lanes S, Sacks ST. The reporting odds ratio and its advantages over the proportional reporting ratio. *Pharmacoepidemiology and Drug Safety*, 2004, 13(8):519-23.

34. Waller P et al. The reporting odds ratio versus the proportional reporting ratio: deuce. *Pharmacoepidemiology and Drug Safety*, 2004, 13(8):525-26.

35. Gogolak V. The effects of backgrounds in safety analysis: the impact of comparison cases on what you see. *Pharmacoepidemiology and Drug Safety*, 2003, 12:249-252.

36. Hauben M, Patadia VK, Goldmsith D. What counts in data mining? *Drug Safety*, 2006, 29(10):827-32.

37. Data mining in spontaneous reports. *Basic and Clinical Pharmacology & Toxicology*, 2006, 98(3):324-330.

38. Personal communication, SJW Evans.

39. Moore N, Thiessard F, Begaud B. The history of disproportionality measures (reporting odds ratio, proportional reporting rates) in spontaneous reporting of adverse drug reactions. *Pharmacoepidemiology and Drug Safety*, 2005, 14:285-286.

40. Hauben M et al. The role of data mining in pharmacovigilance. *Expert Opinion on Drug Safety*, 2005, 4(5):929-948.

41. Hauben M, Bate A. Data mining in drug safety. In Aronson JK (ed). *Side effects of drugs annual 29*. Amsterdam: Elsevier Science Ltd., 2007, xxxiii-xlvi.

42. Chan KA, Hauben M. Signal detection in pharmacovigilance: empirical evaluation of data mining tools. *Pharmacoepidemiology and Drug Safety*, 2005, 14(9):597-99.

43. Hochberg AM, Hauben M. Time-to-signal comparison for drug safety data mining algorithms vs traditional signalling criteria. *Clin Pharmacol Therapy*, 2009, 85(6):600-606.

44. Hauben M, Reich L. Safety-related drug-labelling changes: findings from two data mining algorithms. *Drug Safety*, 2004, 27(10):735-744.

45. Hauben M, Reich L. Drug-induced pancreatitis: lessons in data mining. *British Journal of Clinical Pharmacology*, 2004, 58(5):560-62.

46. Hauben M. Application of an empiric Bayesian data mining algorithm to reports of pancreatitis associated with atypical anti-psychotics. *Pharmacotherapy*, 2004, 24(9):1122-29.

47. Hauben M. Trimethoprim-induced hyperkalemia – lessons in data mining. *British Journal of Clinical Pharmacology*, 2004, 58(3):338-339.

48. Hauben M. Early postmarketing surveillance: data mining points to consider. *Ann Pharmacotherapy*, 2004, 38(10):1625-1630.

49. Roux E et al. Evaluation of statistical association measures for the automatic signal generation in pharmacovigilance. *IEEE Transactions on Information Technology in Biomedicine*, 2005, 9(4):518-27.

50. Roux E et al. Spontaneous reporting system modelling for the evaluation of automatic signal generation methods in pharmacovigilance. In *Advances in statistical methods for the health sciences,* Boston: Birkhauser, 2007.

51. Rolka H et al. Using simulation to assess the sensitivity and specificity of a signal detection tool for multidimensional public health surveillance data. *Statistics in Medicine*, 2005, 24(4):551-562.

52. Matsushita Y et al. Criteria revision and performance comparison of three methods of signal detection applied to the spontaneous reporting database of a pharmaceutical manufacturer. *Drug Safety*, 2007, 30(8):715-726.

53. Hochberg AM et al. An evaluation of three signal detection algorithms using a highly inclusive reference data base. *Drug Safety*, 2009, 32(6):509-25.

54. Hauben M, Reich L. Reply: The evaluation of data mining methods for the simultaneous and systematic detection of safety signal in large databases: lessons to be learned. *Br J Clin Pharmacol,* 2006, 61(1):115-17.

55. Cesana M et al. Bayesian data mining techniques: the evidence provided by signals detected in single-company spontaneous reports databases. *?? ??*

56. Hammond IW et al. Database size and power to detect safety signals in pharmacovigilance. *Expert Opinion on Drug Safety*, 2007, 6(6):713-21.

57. Czarnecki A, Voss S. Safety signals using proportional reporting ratios from company and regulatory databases. *Drug Information Journal*, 2008, 42: 205-210.

58. Hopstadius J et al. Impact of stratification on adverse drug reaction surveillance. *Drug Safety*, 2008; 31(11):1035-48.

59. Evans SJW. Stratification for spontaneous report databases. *Drug Safety*, 2008, 31(11): 1049-52.

60. Hopstadius J et al. Stratification for spontaneous report databases. *Drug Safety*, 2008, 31(12):1146-47.

61. Henegar C et al. Building an ontology of adverse drug reactions for automated signal generation in pharmacovigilance. *Computers in Biology and Medicine*, 2006; 36:748-767.

62. Pearson RK et al. Influence of the MedDRA hierarchy on pharmacovigilance data mining results. *International Journal of Medical Informatics*, 2009 (in press).

63. Hauben M et al. Data mining in pharmacovigilance: computational cost as a neglected performance parameter. *International Journal of Pharmaceutical Medicine*, 2007, 21(5):319-23.

64. Hauben M, Reich L. Potential utility of data-mining algorithms for early detection of potentially fatal/disabling adverse drug reactions: a retrospective evaluation. *Journal of Clinical Pharmacology*, 2005, 45(4):378-84.

65. Guideline 22 – Commentary in International Ethical Guidelines for Epidemiological Studies. CIOMS, Geneva, 2009, pp. 88-89.

66. *Annals of Internal Medicine*, 2004: 141(1): 73-74.

67. Banks D et al. Comparing data mining methods on the VAERS database. *Pharmacoepidemiology and Drug Safety*, 2005, 14:601-609.

VIII

How to develop a signal detection strategy

a. Stakeholder perspectives

In evaluating the optimal design and delivery of a pharmacovigilance system to support a desirable signal detection strategy, it is informative to consider the expectations of stakeholders. These stakeholders fall into four broad categories: 1) consumers; 2) prescribers; 3) government regulators; and 4) pharmaceutical companies (sponsors). The expectations of each are summarized below.

(1) Expectations of consumers

Consumers bring to the regulatory processes several expectations that at first glance appear entirely reasonable but that, in practice, have proven hard to meet for both industry and regulators. These expectations can be summarised as:

- Any drug approved by a regulatory agency should be 100% safe and effective;
- If a drug has a safety problem, this should be declared on the container label and/or packaging; and
- There should not be quality control problems in the manufacturing process which compromise safety or interrupt the product supply chain.

In addition, in some cases there is an expectation that the company/manufacturer is obliged to provide resources towards medical management of any problems that arise from use of the medicine, and/or compensation for any injury.

There has been growing interest and acceptance of the legitimate role of consumers in shaping health policy and processes. In response, regulators around the world are increasingly re-examining their preconceptions regarding the expectations of consumers as they acknowledge the role of consumers as key stakeholders in the pharmacovigilance process. Consequently, several attempts have been made to address consumers' concerns regarding medicines safety to date. Initiatives such as Australia's provision of Consumer Medicine Information (CMI) brochures or the FDA's Med Guide program have sought to educate the public and media about the risks of the products they purchase or are prescribed.

Increased awareness by consumers has an impact on safety information being subjected to signal detection (e.g. the increased number of adverse event reports from consumers). The decision by FDA in 2008 to publish drug safety signals regularly has focused public attention as never before.

(2)   Expectations of prescribers

In general, prescribers expect that:

- Their clinical observation of a safety issue will be properly documented by the company, promptly copied to the regulatory agency and acted upon as necessary;
- Regulatory authorities monitor all products to ensure that any change in benefit-risk is transparently communicated;
- Timely notice of any new significant safety issues not previously included in the product information (PI) e.g. by Dear Doctor/Healthcare Professional letter, etc.;
- Updated product information will be readily available and company sales representatives provide accurate and current product information that is presented in full compliance with regulatory standards;
- As with consumers, access is available to a company employee who can provide specific information in response to a request.

(3)   Expectations of government regulators

Governments usually carry out their responsibility for continually monitoring the safety of drugs in their countries through specialised, administrative agencies which are, typically, a national or local health authority. Governments also expect these regulatory agencies to be objective, fair and competent in their assessment of safety information for medicinal products. The regulatory role includes operation of robust monitoring systems capable of prompt detection of signals of drug safety issues for the products on their market.

Regulatory authorities expect pharmaceutical companies to:

- Behave responsibly, ethically and in compliance with national laws and directives;
- Provide all relevant information when a new drug application is submitted;
- Promptly report any change in benefit:risk as a result of new safety data;
- Provide product information that accurately reflects what is known to date and that supports the safe use of the product.

(4)   Expectations for pharmaceutical companies (sponsors)

Sponsor companies are generally expected by regulators, consumers and prescribers to:

- Maintain an appropriately resourced, quality system for pharmacovigilance;
- Promptly notify the regulatory agency of any new safety concern and take appropriate action (amendments to the product information, letters to prescribers, product recall, etc.);
- Continually evaluate products for adverse effects in special populations, overdose and drug abuse;
- Screen data for potential manufacturing problems through assessment of product complaints;

- Employ a named, identifiable individual (together with contact details) as their designated person responsible for pharmacovigilance of the company's products (in some jurisdictions);

- Promptly notify all concerned regulatory authorities about any significant regulatory action related to product safety in other jurisdictions.

The operational model for a quality pharmacovigilance system requires coherent, transparent processes that are auditable. The adherence by companies to these expectations is important for ensuring public confidence in the regulatory system, the company, and the product (1).

b. Regulatory considerations and international guidance

In many jurisdictions, the pharmacovigilance regulations governing product surveillance are organized according to the registration status of the medicinal product. This dichotomy between pre-approval and post-approval status of a product reflects the availability, quantity and quality of data about safe human use and has significant methodological implications for the choice of tools and data sets to be used in any signal detection program. While the ICH guidelines have, to a large extent, provided some standardization to individual adverse event reporting schemes, there has been little consensus among industry, regulators or the academic community about the exact nature and extent of a model signal detection program that is capable of functioning across an entire medicinal product lifecycle. Nonetheless, a brief review of some of the key guidance and regulations is insightful.

(1) Pre-marketing signal detection

An important differentiating factor in signal detection for a medicinal product prior to approval is the availability of precise denominator data and the ability to compare adverse event incidence rates between two or more carefully selected populations thanks to structured data collection under strictly controlled conditions in accordance with Good Clinical Practice (2). The blinding of investigators and study subjects to therapy assignment in randomized controlled studies also helps reduce bias in ascertaining adverse events. This is in stark contrast to spontaneous reporting systems which rely on third parties to identify and report safety information potentially related to medicinal products.

A detailed discussion of evaluating safety from clinical trials, and hence the identification of emerging safety signals, appears in the report of CIOMS Working Group VI (Management of Safety Information from Clinical Trials) (3). CIOMS VI recognizes the following key sources of new safety information: i) Evaluation of serious individual case safety reports; ii) Periodic aggregate assessment of available clinical safety data (including clinical adverse events and laboratory parameters) without regard to seriousness or causality; and iii) Evaluation of unblinded studies including individual study results and pooled analyses where appropriate. It also emphasizes the need to apply clinical judgment in signal detection. CIOMS Working Group VII developed a guideline for harmonized periodic safety reports for medicinal products in clinical development (4).

(2) Post-marketing surveillance

Regulations in most jurisdictions do not yet specifically address individual case reporting within the context of signal detection and data mining. In applying statistical data mining methods, it should be recognized that individual case safety report data in a given spontaneous reporting database reflects the local and regional requirements for individual case reportability. A basic understanding of the contents and inherent biases of the database being analyzed is essential to proper interpretation of statistical data mining results.

From the global perspective, several ICH documents are relevant to the detection and evaluation of safety signals in the post-marketing environment. ICH guidelines E2C (Clinical safety data management: periodic safety update reports for marketed products) (5) and E2D (Post-approval safety data management: definitions and standards for expedited reporting) (6) provide a technical framework for the requirements of a pharmacovigilance program and a mechanism for the reporting and evaluation of safety information to health authorities globally. ICH guideline E2E (Pharmacovigilance planning) (7) describes the expectations of a routine pharmacovigilance program and clearly includes a requirement for the "continuous monitoring of the safety profile of approved products including signal detection, issue evaluation, updating of labelling, and liaison with regulatory authorities." The Annex to ICH E2E also describes the role of data mining as adjunctive to the role of analyses of single case reports.

In the European Union (EU), Volume 9A of the Rules Governing Medicinal Products in the European Union (8) provides guidelines for the interpretation and implementation of pharmacovigilance within the EU legal framework. Relevant to the application of statistical data mining methods, the EudraVigilance Expert Working Group of the EMA has issued a guideline on the use of statistical signal detection methods in the EudraVigilance Data Analysis System (9).

The FDA Guidance on Good Pharmacovigilance Practices and Pharmacoepidemiology Assessment (10) also provides an overview of data mining methods while stating explicitly that a formal data mining program is not mandatory for a signal detection program. The guidance also places data mining approaches in the context of an integrated signal detection program with other pharmacovigilance methods, such as case series evaluation and determination of reporting rates and incidence rates.

c. Value added for integrating data mining methods into a signal detection program

Given the limitations of spontaneous report data (see Chapter IV) and statistical data mining methods (see Chapter VII), it is important that the organization contemplating the integration of data mining approaches into a comprehensive pharmacovigilance program sets clearly defined operational objectives and plans for the organizational changes and additional resources that would be required.

A number of reports have described the retrospective application of statistical data mining algorithms to evaluate if known adverse drug reactions might have been detected earlier, usually relative to the timing of a regulatory action taken (e.g. changes to prescribing information and product withdrawal). The results of these retrospective evaluations have been mixed, with some authors reporting that conventional procedures identify most associations earlier than data mining algorithms (*11*) while others report the opposite (*12*). However, little is known about the predictive validity of the currently available statistical data mining methods as applied prospectively. This should not be interpreted to indicate that statistical data mining methods are not useful. Rather, it suggests that the most realistic view would fall somewhere between the extremes of "unbridled optimism" and "considerable pessimism" noted by Bate and Edwards (*13*) and that both the strengths and weakness of these methods should be carefully considered.

A further consideration should be given to the matter of potential conflicts of interest when reviewing the data mining literature. With an increasing web of relationships between data mining software vendors, regulatory authorities and pharmaceutical companies, competing interests should be fully and openly declared. Some of these competing interests are linked to commercial and intellectual ownership of specific data mining algorithms.

The incremental value of statistical data mining methods as an adjunct to a comprehensive pharmacovigilance program is ultimately dependent on the organization's careful assessment of potential gains versus potential limitations. Practical implications of systematically adopting data mining approaches should also be taken into consideration (see sections d and e below). Despite the challenges in scientifically assessing the incremental value, systematically collected signal detection metrics would help evaluate the efficiency and effectiveness of the signal detection methods as a part of a comprehensive pharmacovigilance program.

d. Practical, technical and strategic points to consider

When it comes to the design and execution of a signal detection program, there is no such a thing as "one size fits all" and therefore a single piece of universal prescriptive advice cannot be provided as to how to integrate statistical data mining approaches into an overall signal detection program. The reader is advised to consider the following points in making a decision on the practical, technical, and strategic aspects of their signal detection program. Decisions will be influenced by the situation, ranging from a regulatory authority responsible for monitoring the safety of all medicines on the market, to an individual company introducing a new medicine to a number of markets.

(1) Selection of data types and sources

Publicly accessible spontaneous adverse event report data

Regulatory authorities and international monitoring centres typically have their own signal detection programs to detect safety signals that may have an impact on the safety of patients in their respective geopolitical territories. Marketing authorization holders (MAHs) may consider including a publicly accessible section of adverse event databases, most notably WHO's Vigibase and the United States FDA's AERS database, in their signal detection program to:

- Identify adverse event reports that have been reported directly to regulatory authorities but not to the MAH;

- Perform disproportionality and other statistical analyses to examine the characteristics of adverse event reports associated with the MAH's product in comparison with those associated with other products in the same pharmacological class. This would be particularly helpful when the MAH's internal safety database cannot provide a robust reference dataset due to the limited number or diversity of products and adverse event data represented.

Company spontaneous adverse event report data

The MAH may consider applying advanced data mining techniques to its own adverse event report database (company safety database), which they maintain to comply with regulatory obligations for reviewing, and submit individual case safety reports (ICSRs) and periodic safety update reports (PSURs) according to applicable national and regional requirements (*see 3 and 4*). The MAH should consider the following points before designing a data mining program using a company safety database:

- The company database may be too small or too specialized (e.g. overrepresentation of one therapeutic area or adverse events known to be related to a specific product);

- Data in a company database may be subject to a bias in reporting frequency of a specific drug-event combination due to various factors affecting reporting behaviour, such as heightened awareness of a specific drug-event combination (e.g. media coverage, notable changes in prescribing information) and time on the market (e.g. the Weber effect: higher reporting rates in the first two years of marketing followed by decreasing trends).

Clinical trial data

Clinical trial data are given heavier weight during the development phase in a product's life cycle. Well-designed randomized controlled trials provide high quality adverse event data, which could indicate an imbalance of adverse event risk between treated and untreated subjects. Even though relative weights of clinical trial data in an overall signal detection program tend to decrease as the post-marketing experience increases, post-approval studies with specific safety endpoints should be considered, when appropriate, as a part of safety monitoring and risk management plans. Principles and practical recommendations for signal detection with clinical trial data have been addressed in the report of the CIOMS Working Group VI (*see 3*).

Other data sources

Not all data sources discussed below and in Chapter V may be easily accessible to those considering their use because of the confidential and proprietary nature of the data. Value added for analyzing additional data in a given signal detection program must be evaluated against the costs and efforts required to obtain access.

An increasing number of healthcare data sources (e.g. medical records and insurance claims) are now maintained electronically. Some of these data are available for pharmacoepidemiological studies and safety monitoring, mostly to address specific research questions or targeted safety issues. Typical epidemiological and pharmacovigilance considerations are:

- Is the question reasonably well refined to be translated into a concrete study or monitoring plan? How would a study population and endpoint of interest be defined?

- Does the database under consideration contain information suitable to address the question at hand with respect to patient populations, product usage patterns, etc.?

- Does the database provide an adequate sample size?

- What ethical and privacy issues need to be considered?

- What value would the use of specific data sources or types and analytical methods add to a better understanding of a given safety issue? The value cannot be judged on its own without considering what other methods are used to complement the limitations of the method under consideration (14).

(2) Attributes of the data

When developing and executing a signal detection program, a through understanding of the databases (data sources) used is needed, including the strengths and weaknesses of the data selected for signal detection purposes; e.g. the size of the database and the types of drugs included, coding conventions, and the level of evidence available.

Data volume – size of dataset

- *Small volume*: Consider expert clinical review, supported by triage algorithms to partition data and prioritize work, automated cross reference to core clinical safety information (or other references, such as the Summary of Product Characteristics and package leaflets) and automated literature reference sources.

- *Large volume*: Add data mining as a way of screening large volumes of data. Most data mining methods are based on the concept of disproportionality. Within limits, all measures of disproportionality are basically similar, but:
  - ❑ When the background (reference drug group) is narrow in scope (few drug products or specialized "niche" products), the result will be less reflective of general reporting. Sometimes this is helpful (as when comparing drugs in the same class and user population, e.g. vaccines), sometimes less so.
  - ❑ Because the method depends on estimates of disproportional reporting, if the reporting fraction is variable or has strong biases in reporting, signals may be hidden (but the obvious ones accentuated).
  - ❑ Stratification can obscure some signals and artificially accentuate others, particularly where there are small strata. Triage should provide an analysis of important variables.

All these limitations become more important the smaller the dataset.

Data quality

Safety data commonly used for signal detection often have their own quality assurance and quality control procedures. For instance, a safety database containing individual case safety report (ICSR) data should be subject to rigorous system validation requirements and adequate staff training to comply with local, regional, and global standards. However, the quality standards and database architecture sufficient for ICSR processing and submission may not be optimal when the data are used for aggregate analysis and data mining. Furthermore, the chances of obtaining additional information on reported cases are highest at the time of initial reporting and immediate follow up, and therefore the importance of due diligence in collecting data for signal detection purposes must be well understood by the staff responsible for initial case intake and processing. Key points to consider include:

- Data cleansing and quality assurance of all steps from the original reporter to the output from the database are essential (*15*).

- Software that prompts and supports data input is highly advantageous.

- Automated coding can easily lead to information being lost and has a potential for miscoding of the free text. How terms are lumped or split must be transparent and tested in a contingency fashion.

- Data mining cannot improve data quality though it is robust and exposes missing data and can be used for duplicate detection, and cluster analysis (sometimes useful to detect errors and fraud).

- The quality of data (e.g. completeness of information in spontaneous adverse event reports) may be scored systematically and presented in analysis. However, no data should ever be excluded from an analysis for signal detection automatically without justification. A report of poor quality may nevertheless represent a valid case for an emerging signal. The use of a standard questionnaire will help to collect information systematically and consistently.

- Possible confounders that could provide alternative explanations of the results:
  - ❏ Factors that affect reporting behaviour and thus the reporting trends observed; stimulated reporting (heightened awareness)
  - ❏ Time on the market: a drug that recently came to market should not be compared with a product that has been on the market for a long time. Appropriate time windows for analysis should be chosen
  - ❏ Choice of a comparison (reference) group: the entire database excluding the drug of interest versus restriction to patients receiving specific drug groups (e.g. transplant patients receiving another immunosuppressant drug).

Data dictionaries, coding and query tools

The ability to extract data from the database in consistent fashion is critical. How adverse event report data are entered into a database will have an impact on the efficiency and adequacy of data extraction, processing, and analysis for signal detection purposes (*16, 17, 18*). Often a safety database is designed and configured to optimize the efficiency of processing individual case safety reports (ICSRs) and accommodate the most recent regulatory requirements for ICSR submission. This may result in a lack of consistency in data dictionary versions and coding conventions over time. Attention should be paid to the following data fields among others:

- *Adverse event (reaction) term:* Most safety databases use the Medical Dictionary for Regulatory Activities (MedDRA). The history of dictionary version changes should be considered in defining case search criteria, whether one MedDRA preferred term (PT), a group of MedDRA PTs (e.g. Standard MedDRA Queries or SMQs), or other groupings of MedDRA terms from various hierarchy levels.

- *Product name:* Both generic (chemical) and proprietary (brand) names should be included when applicable. Some drugs may have multiple brand names that are used in different geographic regions. It may be difficult to attribute a product to a specific manufacturer when generic or biosimilar products are available and the reporter of adverse events cannot distinguish between them.

- *Report origin:* This is important when stratifying analysis by the origin of adverse event reports; e.g. clinical study versus post-marketing spontaneous reporting.

- *Date and other quantitative values:* Date format and units of laboratory test results must be consistent or standardized.

- For identifying a series of cases to address a particular safety issue, adverse event coding and other data entry conventions should be optimal

- The safety database structure should facilitate the extraction, simple tabulation, and advanced statistical analysis of data.

(3) Attributes of drugs under monitoring

Therapeutic or pharmacological class

If the product under monitoring is in a therapeutic or pharmacological class with known or suspected safety issues, a signal detection program for the product should incorporate methods for identifying and analyzing relevant cases in timely fashion. Clinical or observational studies to address those safety concerns may be warranted.

Product life cycle and time on market

The weights attached to various data sources and analytical methods will change over time:

- *Immediately after the initial product launch:* There is heavy reliance on safety data from clinical trials. If the product becomes widely used rapidly, sentinel cases of an adverse reaction that were not observed during clinical trials may start to arise. Safety issues associated with product usage patterns in the real-world setting may become manifest. The assessment of initial spontaneous adverse event report data tends to focus on individual case review or case series analysis rather than the application of advanced statistical methods;

- *Several years after the initial product launch:* The weights placed on post-marketing safety data for rare events and events with longer latency will gradually increase. Long-term observational studies may be considered for structured and targeted data collection to address specific safety concerns. Clinical trials will continue to be a valuable source of new safety information if expanded or new indications are pursued for the product;
- *Many years after the product launch:* The chances of detecting new safety information will decrease as the product matures and its safety profile becomes established. However, there are well-known examples of detection of safety signals many years after marketing, e.g. pure red cell aplasia associated with erythropoietins.

(4) Attributes of patient populations under monitoring

A signal detection program for a specific product needs to consider the demographic and clinical characteristics of the patient populations being treated that gave rise to the cases, as well as the characteristics of populations that are used as comparison groups. When interpreting the results, the incidence and prevalence of the adverse event in the treated population need to be considered and sources of reliable background rate data consulted.

Underlying conditions and risk factors

The observed association may be due to the indication for therapy rather than the therapy itself (e.g. if a positive PRR for renal failure is obtained in renal transplant patients, the incidence of renal failure in this patient group needs to be addressed). The following variables should also be considered:
- Co-morbid conditions
- Concomitant medicine use
- Risk factors for the adverse events observed.

Demographics

The following variables are commonly considered in a safety data analysis:
- Gender
- Age
- Race/ethnicity
- Geographic distribution.

Stratification of analysis by these variables may be warranted when it is suspected that an adverse effect of the medicinal product may vary across different demographic groups. Almenoff et al. (2007) (*19*) has presented an example of applying disproportionality analysis to explore the possible demographic effects in subpopulations.

(5) Choosing specifications for a quantitative signalling approach

A technical discussion of various data sources and statistical methods is provided in Chapter VII. When designing a signal detection program with quantitative methods, the points described below should be considered. No matter what choices are made, the methods used in a quantitative signal detection approach must be clearly documented to ensure appropriate interpretation of generated signals and facilitate the planning of subsequent investigations.

Selection of statistical methods

The statistical methods used must be compatible with the data sources selected. Statistical methods for safety signal detection are often developed for application to certain data types. For example, statistical methods for disproportionality analysis have been developed specifically to analyse spontaneous adverse event data for which reliable patient exposure data (denominators) are not available. The advantages and limitations associated with various disproportionality analysis methods must be recognized. In some circumstances it may be preferable to use more than one method. Stratification and other modifications to analytic methods should be considered when adjustments for selected covariates (e.g. gender, age group, geographic region, and time to onset) are likely to increase the sensitivity and/or specificity of statistical analysis. These adjustments could be applied at the initial screening phase or subsequent to triage of initial screening results, depending on the characteristics of treated populations and potential safety concerns. Regardless of the method selected, thorough piloting should be undertaken prior to introduction.

Limitations inherent in statistical methods and associated assumptions

Over-representation of a specific drug-event association in the comparator group: if there is a strong association between the event or event group under investigation and a drug in a reference (comparison) group, disproportionality analysis is likely to lead to a false negative result for any other drug examined regarding this event or event group. For example, if drug X accounts for 60% of agranulocytosis cases in the database but for only 10% of the case volume, leaving this drug in the comparison group is likely to produce non-significant disproportionality scores for agranulocytosis for any other drug tested against the remaining database. Excluding drug X from the comparison group leads to higher sensitivity of the method of identifying agranulocytosis as a safety signal for other drugs.

Event group definition is too broad and includes non-specific terms: if not just one PT, but a group of PTs (event group, such as a Standard MedDRA Query or SMQ) is used to generate disproportionality scores, the inclusion of non-specific PTs in the event group definition may lead to false negative results. For instance, if the event group definition for neuroleptic malignant syndrome for drug Y includes PT "pyrexia" in addition to PTs "neuroleptic malignant syndrome" and "malignant hyperthermia," a disproportionality score may be non-significant due to the decreased specificity in the event group definition. This is often a dilemma, however, as the exact nature and extent of a safety issue may not be clearly definable with limited information when the issue is initially emerging.

Thresholds and other rules for filtering and triaging data mining results

Data mining methods, as an initial screening tool, inevitably generate some false positive and false negative results, the frequency of which will be dictated by the sensitivity and specificity of the methods and operationally determined by thresholds and other triage rules (see Chapter VII for technical discussions of specific statistical algorithms and associated thresholds found in published literature). The optimal level of a trade-off between false positive and false negative results will vary across different organizations, depending on the following:

- The place of data mining within the context of an overall signal detection program, depending on what other approaches are used to complement the data mining approach.

- The characteristics of different datasets, which affect the choice of optimal methodology. For example, a small company safety database may have detailed case information including narratives, and ease of access to the original reporter for additional data collection as required, but is likely to lack the size and diversity needed for analysis with disproportionality tools. In contrast, WHO's Vigibase and FDA's AERS databases contain more limited case information, but contain four decades' worth of data on thousands of marketed products. As these two types of datasets are likely to be used for different operational objectives, optimal rules for data mining (i.e. the particular statistic used and thresholds chosen) may differ.

Statistical thresholds can be modified depending on the clinical situation, stage in lifecycle of the medicine, availability of other methodologies etc., as well as the false positive/false negative trade-off.

Frequency of analysis

Signal detection is an ongoing systematic process, and data mining and other quantitative analysis must be performed regularly and periodically. The following points should be considered when scheduling data mining runs and other analyses. A single signal detection program is expected to have various analysis components with different frequencies of execution.

- The volume of new adverse event report information gained per unit time: a fast growing dataset may warrant more frequent analysis in general.

- The type of adverse reaction: reports of rare events, particularly those which are serious or not observed previously, may need to be recognized by pharmacovigilance staff immediately after the reports are received. In contrast, reports for more common events and known adverse reactions may be better analyzed at the aggregate level at a prescheduled frequency.

- Overall process efficiency: initial analysis and data mining runs, as well as subsequent investigations, may be scheduled to optimize their linkage to other pharmacovigilance processes and milestone events; e.g. the production of periodic safety update reports, the completion of major safety studies, a risk management plan or a risk minimization plan.

Use of patient exposure (denominator) data

Disproportionality analysis has been developed for examining spontaneous case report data, which does not permit absolute risk (e.g. incidence rates) of a given adverse event to be estimated. The availability of patient exposure data aids in assessing time trends of adverse event reporting. However, the limitations of both numerators (case counts) and denominators (exposure) must be well recognized in the interpretation of reporting rates, particularly taking into account the known variable degree of under-reporting (20). Application of inferential statistics (e.g. confidence limits and p-values) to the analysis of reporting rates is therefore not advisable.

e. Operational model and organizational infrastructure

(1) Guiding principles

The following guiding principles should be considered in establishing and maintaining a pharmacovigilance program. These are applicable to programs for both sponsors (i.e. companies) and regulatory authorities:

- Pharmacovigilance organizations should work within an *operating model* that is designed to support the core responsibilities of a pharmacovigilance unit. The model should coordinate and align pharmacovigilance activities across relevant business units; it should facilitate rapid, informed communication and decision-making for the protection of patient safety;

- Pharmacovigilance organizations need *tools and processes* to optimize the detection and evaluation of safety signals. Staff should be trained and these training activities documented;

- Staff working within this operating model require an *organizational infrastructure* that supports holistic monitoring of product safety throughout the product lifecycle (i.e. development through launch and post-marketing phases). This is most efficiently accomplished when pharmacovigilance staff members routinely collaborate with experts from different functions, such as clinical development, statistics, clinical pharmacology, toxicology, epidemiology, and outcomes research. One efficient way to accomplish this is through the establishment of product or therapeutic area matrix teams, where constituents from some or all of these disciplines, depending on the needs of the program, meet on a periodic basis (21);

- Pharmacovigilance activities and decision-making vis-à-vis product safety need to be transparent, consistent across organizations and in compliance with both corporate SOPs and legal requirements. For companies, these activities are subject to regulatory audit (see below).

(2) Design and implementation of data management systems

Legal and regulatory requirements for pharmacovigilance systems

The organization may be subject to very specific legal and regulatory requirements covering both pre- and post-authorization safety monitoring. These requirements may have a direct impact on the technical choice for the data mining or signal detection system and its interface with the underlying pharmacovigilance database.

In addition, the organization may need to comply with local technical standards, which may be applicable to the storage and exchange of electronic records including pharmacovigilance information (e.g. Title 21 Code of Federal Regulations Part 11 (*22*) and the EU Privacy Directives and Policies on Exchange of Data across Borders (*23*)). The system requirements must also take into account the local requirements for data confidentiality and data protection (i.e. personal data protection and the commercial nature of the information) and ensure that these are not violated during implementation or use of the signal detection system.

Resources and business requirements

The business requirements should be clearly established before commencing software or system development. These requirements should take into consideration the following, among other elements:

- The volume and complexity of safety information to be handled and analyzed;

- The resources available (financial and human resources, which must and can be allocated to the development, implementation, validation and maintenance of the system) taking into account the business requirements:
  - ❏ A thorough evaluation of these resources, considering different options for technical solutions (e.g. an off-the-shelf database versus in-house development; in-house use versus outsourcing), is recommended before any technical choice is made;
  - ❏ Some organizations have procurement procedures to comply with, which require long-term planning of the system's requirements, costs, resources and deliverables.

- The structure of the organization, users' management and registration, access to the information, and security:
  - ❏ Consideration should be given to whether access is needed at a single location or in numerous geographical regions such as affiliates or regional pharmacovigilance centres;
  - ❏ The definition of the users' rights is crucial and the system must be developed to accommodate different levels of access and support the relevant security functionalities.

- Other technical and operational considerations, such as:
  - ❏ Integration with the existing IT infrastructure;
  - ❏ Availability of a back-up or business continuity system;
  - ❏ Resources and costs for customization work required for an off-the-shelf product as well as maintenance and evolution of the system (e.g. system upgrades).

User interactions with the system

It is important to optimize the way that users interface with the systems that are available to them. Ease of use will likely correlate with both the acceptance and utilization of the system by the users. Optimal utilization of the system will in turn help ensure the effective pharmacovigilance activities for an organization's product portfolio (*24*) or national marketing authorization range.

It is important to avoid a mismatch between the needs of users and the complexity and resources required to manage the system:

- In order to minimize costs and risks, it is recommended that a comprehensive list of user requirements be established and shared with prospective stakeholders before commencing any system design work;

- It is also very important that key user groups/stakeholders continue to work closely with IT system designers throughout the development phase to ensure user needs are met;

- Training needs for both technical support staff and business users need to be carefully considered and planned.

Options for system specification choice

A system must be chosen based on its ability to handle the anticipated workload and data volume. Software and hardware must be able to handle the requirements of a signal detection algorithm, work at a practical speed, and give valid results. However, if the hardware is unable to handle the demands of a sophisticated software program working on a large database, alternative approaches may need to be taken; e.g.:

- Adjust the signal detection algorithm, so that the work can be handled within a realistic timeframe by the hardware available; e.g. computationally demanding Bayesian methods may need to be replaced with simple proportional reporting ratios;

- Run computationally demanding algorithms when the system usage is low (e.g. during the evening) or in a parallel computing system, and then make the results of the calculations available to users periodically (e.g. monthly).

Project management

The technical implementation should follow a strict and detailed project plan based on the definition of the business requirements and technical specifications. Such a plan will maximize the chances of achieving a correct technical implementation of the specifications with limited delay, even in the face of unforeseeable challenges.

The plan should also consider non-IT aspects, which will have an impact on the conduct and success of the project; e.g.:

- Procedures that the organization should follow during the technical implementation of the system (e.g. public procurement procedures or internal financial procedures). If some work is outsourced, the project management plan needs be tied to the contractual agreement(s) between the different parties involved in the project implementation;

- Preparation and deployment of user training materials.

Technical implementation must be monitored by a multidisciplinary project management team, with project management resources allotted:

- Good communication within the project development team, particularly that between the business and technical stakeholders, is crucial;

- Decision-making authority and issue escalation processes should be made clear among all stakeholders.

Testing and validation

Any new system must undergo appropriate validation and testing:
- When the system uses a new algorithm, both the system and algorithm must undergo stringent validation and testing;
- Even if a commercial software product is purchased, it is important to perform some validation of the tools and a "sense check" of system outputs by comparing results obtained "in house" with data in published literature or with well established product knowledge such as the product label;
- For some algorithms, results can be validated by comparing them to calculations made outside of the system.

If the data mining algorithm is to be applied within the adverse event database, it is important to establish that operation of the software program on the database does not violate the integrity of the data in the database.

Any changes to the system, algorithm, or other technical methods must be re-tested and managed through appropriate change control processes.

f. Quality assurance for the signal detection program

(1) Guiding principles

The value added by applying quantitative data mining methods must be assessed within the context of an overall, comprehensive signal detection program. Therefore, a decision to employ quantitative approaches, no matter what data sources and statistical methods are chosen, should be made by careful assessment of: 1) other methods used, and 2) the availability of additional data.

Even if various program components and source data have met validation and quality criteria, the quality of an overall signal detection program needs to be ensured. Particular attention should be paid to the following points:
- The documented qualifications and training of personnel involved in the program;
- The need for clearly defined roles and responsibilities of different functions and staff members, including clearly described hand-off points in the signal detection workflow;
- Consistent good practices in documenting analyses, reviews, and decisions;
- Clear linkage between the signal detection program and the related process e.g. ICSR processing, periodic safety reporting, creating a risk management plan and risk communication.

(2) Measures of effectiveness and efficiency

Many recognized challenges in assessing the effectiveness and efficiency of quantitative signal detection methods are due to the inherent limitations of the signal methods themselves. Key practical points to consider are:

82

- The value of data mining algorithms as an adjunct to a comprehensive pharmacovigilance program is ultimately dependent on the organization's careful assessment of potential gains versus potential disadvantages;

- An organization's adoption of data mining must include clearly defined operational objectives, as well as an understanding of the organizational changes and additional resources required for data mining to be successfully integrated into a comprehensive pharmacovigilance program;

- An evaluation of quantitative signalling methods must take into account not only the method used but also the data analyzed, prior and posterior knowledge and decisions, and any other data processing details;

- The metrics to be measured and evaluated for the signal detection program must be aligned to the objectives of the program; that is, the metrics must have a potential for influencing further operation of the program (e.g. modifications to parameter specifications in statistical methods; changes in the frequency of data review).

Sample metrics

The list below shows sample metrics which could be considered for assessing the operational efficiency and effectiveness of a signal detection program, particularly the value of adding quantitative, data mining methods to an overall signal detection program:

- Total number of signals identified;

- Number and clinical significance (public health impact) of safety signals identified through traditional pharmacovigilance methods versus those of signals identified through data mining;

- Number of safety signals found by regulators versus sponsor;

- Time to signal detection versus other stakeholders;

- Time from signal identification to risk minimization action; this should be stratified by the clinical significance or the public health impact of the signal (e.g. based on impact analysis).

(3) Compliance

Sponsors (companies) have an obligation to comply with all regulations applicable to adverse event reporting and to pharmacovigilance. Additionally, they need to ensure that within their organizations, staff members are compliant with the standard operating procedures (SOPs) of their organizations.

It is prudent for sponsors to conduct internal audits as part of a quality management program to ensure that their company is compliant with both the regulations as well as its own corporate SOPs. Such internal audits not only prepare and educate the sponsor for regulatory inspection processes, but they enable detection of process inadequacies that can be proactively remedied. The British Association of Research Quality Assurance has published a useful guide for pharmacovigilance auditors; this information may also be used for audit preparation by sponsor organizations (*25*).

Audit preparation should also evaluate the information and data flow across various types of activities, to ensure that the processes in place do not have gaps. Such gaps are most likely to exist when specific activities lie across multiple business units; special attention should be paid to operations that involve business units that collaborate in some areas but whose business roles are not directly linked. Examples of these include:

- The absence of a formal link between manufacturing and pharmacovigilance organizations to review and communicate about product complaints;

- Deficits in adverse reporting processes used by small local affiliates and/or licensing partners of a large company.

g. Conclusions and recommendations

No single piece of universal prescriptive advice can be provided to those planning to design and execute a signal detection program as to how to integrate statistical data mining approaches into an overall signal detection program. Instead, the reader is advised to consider a range of practical, technical, and strategic points.

- There has been little consensus so far among industry, regulators or the academic community about the exact nature and extent of a model signal detection program that is capable of functioning across an entire medicinal product lifecycle. Nonetheless, a review of selected key guidance and regulations is insightful.

- Both the strengths and limitations of statistical data mining methods should be carefully considered. The results of retrospective application of statistical data mining algorithms to evaluate if known adverse drug reactions might have been detected earlier have been mixed.

- The organization contemplating the integration of data mining approaches into a comprehensive pharmacovigilance program should set clearly defined operational objectives and plan for the organizational changes and additional resources that would be required.

- Consideration of the expectations of (and for) stakeholders, including consumers, prescribers, government regulators, and pharmaceutical companies (sponsors) is informative in evaluating the optimal design and delivery of a pharmacovigilance system to support a desirable signal detection strategy.

Special guidance for emerging pharmacovigilance regulatory centres

It should be clearly recognized that, despite the interest and energies around technology and the automation of some of the drug surveillance and signal detection programs, the available evidence to support their optimal role in an overall pharmacovigilance program is still evolving.

In those regulatory environments where legislation and processes in the area of signal detection and data mining have not fully been established, the Uppsala Monitoring Centre has a collaborative WHO Program for International Drug Monitoring (26). The integration of pharmacovigilance into a broader scheme of public health is another important consideration in these regions (27).

References

1. MHRA Pharmacovigilance Inspectorate. *Good pharmacovigilance practice.* 2008. (http://www.mhra.gov.uk/Howweregulate/Medicines/Inspectionandstandards/GoodPharmacovigilancePractice/index.htm).

2. ICH Guideline E6 (R1): *Good clinical practice: consolidated guideline.*

3. *Management of safety information from clinical trials.* Report of Working Group VI. Geneva, CIOMS, 2005.

4. *The development safety update report (DSUR): harmonizing the format and content for periodic safety reporting during clinical trials.* Report of Working Group VII. Geneva, CIOMS, 2006.

5. ICH Guideline E2C (R1): *Clinical safety data management: periodic safety update reports for marketed drugs.* 2003.

6. ICH Guideline E2D: *Post-approval safety data management: definitions and standards for expedited reporting.* 2003.

7. ICH Guideline E2E: *Pharmacovigilance planning.* 2004.

8. Eudralex Volume 9A, The *rules governing medicinal products in the European Union.* March 2007.

9. EudraVigilance Expert Working Group. *Guideline on the use of statistical signal detection methods in the EudraVigilance data analysis system.* June 2008.

10. US FDA *Guidance for Industry: Good Pharmacovigilance Practices and Pharmacoepidemiologic Assessment.* March 2005. (http://www.fda.gov/cder/guidance/6359OCC.htm).

11. Lehman HP et al. An evaluation of computer-aided disproportionality analysis for post-marketing signal detection. *Clinical Pharmacology &Therapeutics*, 2007, 82(2):173-80.

12. Szarfman A, Machado S, O'Neill RT. Use of screening algorithms and computer systems to efficiently signal combinations of drugs in the US FDA's spontaneous reports database. *Drug Safety*, 2002, 25(6):381-392.

13. Bate A, Edwards IR. Data mining in spontaneous reports. *Basic Clin Pharmacol Toxicology*, 2006, 98(3):330-35.

14. Ståhl M et al. Introducing triage logic as a new strategy for the detection of signals in the WHO Drug Monitoring database. *Pharmacoepidemiology and Drug Saf*ety, 2004, 13:355-363.

15. Lindquist M. Data quality management in pharmacovigilance. *Drug Safety*, 2004, 27(12):857-70.

16. Bousquet C et al. Implementation of automated signal generation in pharmacovigilance using a knowledge-based approach. *International Journal of Medical Informatics,* 2005, 74:563-571.

17. Purcell PM. Data mining in pharmacovigilance. *International Journal of Pharmaceutical Medicine*, 2003, 17(2): 63-64.

18. Hauben M, Patadia VK, Goldmsith D. What counts in data mining? *Drug Safety*, 2006, 29(10):827-32.

19. Almenoff JS et al. Novel statistical tools for monitoring the safety of marketed drugs. *Clinical Pharmacology &Therapeutics*, 2007, 82(2):157-66.

20. Graham DJ, Ahmad SR, Piazza-Hepp T. Spontaneous Reporting–USA. In: Mann RD and Andrews EB, eds. *Pharmacovigilance.* Chichester, UK, John Wiley & Sons, 2002, pp. 219-227.

21. Brewster W et al. Evolving paradigms in pharmacovigilance. *Current Drug Safety*, 2006, 1, 127-134.

22. Food and Drug Administration, Title 21 *Code of Federal Regulations* (21 CFR Part 11).

23. http://ec.europa.eu/justice home/fsj/privacy/law/index en.htm

24. Hauben M et al. Data mining in pharmacovigilance: computational cost as a neglected performance parameter. *International Journal of Pharmaceutical Medicine,* 2007, 21:319-323.

25. Pharmacovigilance Auditing-A BARQA (British Association of Research Quality Assurance). *Guide for Auditors*. Helen Powell and members of the Good Pharmacovigilance Practice Working Party, 2006.

26. *The importance of pharmacovigilance: safety monitoring of medicinal products*. Geneva, WHO, 2002.

27. *The safety of medicines in public health programmes: pharmacovigilance as an essential tool*. Geneva, WHO, 2006.

IX

Overview of signal management

Signal management consists of a set of activities including signal prioritization and evaluation to determine whether a signal represents a risk which may warrant further assessment, communication or other risk minimization actions in accordance with the public health importance of the issue. Following signal evaluation, a signal either becomes an identified risk, a potential risk (which implies that closer monitoring and/or further investigation is necessary), or does not constitute a risk and does not warrant further action at that time.

When important information about a signal is missing, additional activities designed to address the gaps should be considered. The objective is to investigate the possibility of a risk or to provide reassurance about the absence of a risk. A potential risk would trigger closer monitoring (e.g. questionnaires, active surveillance) and/or further investigation (e.g. epidemiological studies) and may, in selected cases, already warrant precautionary risk communication and minimisation activities at this stage.

For identified risks resulting from a verified signal, risk minimisation activities should always be considered and the risks should continue to be monitored for changes in severity, characteristics or frequency.

When a signal does not constitute a potential or identified risk, it will not require further action except for the need to keep monitoring it via routine pharmacovigilance processes for changes in severity, characteristics, or frequency. Criteria could be set to notify (i.e. alert) safety evaluators (within health authorities and pharmaceutical companies) of such changes.

The starting point for signal management is that nearly all reasoning and decision making take place in the presence of some uncertainty. Information acquisition and criteria for a decision are the two main components of the decision-making process. Acquiring relevant and bias-free information is important as its effect is to increase the likelihood of making a correct decision in the signal management process. The criteria for a decision on whether a signal constitutes a potential or identified risk include using one's own judgment in the process; different decision makers may feel that all types of error are not equal.

In the framework of signal management, the Company Core Safety Information (CSI) constitutes the basic reference against which signals are evaluated. In this respect, a signal should not exclusively be understood as a new adverse finding (i.e. not yet described in the latest CSI) but should include adverse findings which, upon review, have elements that indicate a greater specificity, severity or frequency compared to the wording used in the CSI, or that indicate a medication error.

This chapter addresses each of the above elements in a coherent process incorporating the following three steps (see Figure 1, Chapter III): (a) signal prioritization, (b) signal evaluation (i.e. acquisition of new relevant information) and risk determination, and (c) decision making resulting in subsequent actions as appropriate (e.g. further signal characterization, signal communication). Similar approaches have been reviewed in previous publications (*1*, *2*, *3*). Risk communication and risk minimization are not the detailed subject of the present review.

a. Signal prioritization

Signal prioritization is a first critical step in signal management. Evaluating all signals (i.e. single or aggregated reports) in detail has major resource implications as many will turn out not to be real ("*false alarm*") or alternatively to require action. This is not to say that the signal can be dismissed without some kind of evaluation. The prioritization process implies that all signals will be reviewed but some more expeditiously than others. In this respect, there is general agreement that unexpected serious signals occurring during the first years post-marketing should be looked at as a priority in order to establish as rapidly as possible the safety profile of the compound under evaluation.

System-based platforms have been developed to allow efficient knowledge management of safety signals by integrating simple filtering algorithms, simplifying data retrieval and reducing duplicative work (*4*). At the time of print, there has not been enough experience with any of the available vendor software. As such, the CIOMS Working Group VIII does not recommend any product over another.

(1) Impact analysis

Not all safety signals represent "risks" (i.e. potential or identified) and an initial signal prioritization is required to determine which signals should require immediate attention. Key determinants of risk include the strength of evidence, the medical significance (i.e. the potential for prevention, seriousness, severity, reversibility, and consequence) and the potential impact on public health (i.e. the implication of occurrence in the population at large).

Very few impact analysis approaches have been published. Waller et al. (*8, 9*) have developed and piloted a mathematical scoring system to aid signal prioritization from spontaneous adverse event data. Each score combines quantitative and/or qualitative criteria. The evidence score (from 1 to 100) for an event and a drug of interest is obtained by multiplying a PRR/95% CI score by a second score quantifying the strength of evidence of a single case/case series by a third score for the biological plausibility of the event reported with the drug of interest. The public health score (from 1 to 100) is based on the number of cases reported per year, the health consequence and the reporting rate. Plotting the evidence score versus the public health score identifies four categories of attention with different consequential actions. Because inputs are subjective or subject to random error, it is recommended to perform a sensitivity analysis (*see 8*).

Table 9 summarizes the points that may be considered for initial signal prioritization, the most rudimentary being to focus on serious unexpected signals. Based on these determinants, signals with potential high impact require immediate attention and an expedited evaluation. The purpose of an impact analysis is to guide medical judgment, to reduce subjectivity and to allocate resources proportionate to risk.

Table 9: Points to consider for initial signal prioritization, not in hierarchical order (see *5, 6, 7*)

- New (not yet reported) adverse reaction
- Serious*
- Medically significant (e.g. severe, irreversible, lead to an increased morbidity or mortality, list of "critical terms" or "Designated Medical Events")
- Presence in a "drug-specific" list of surveillance terms (i.e. a limited list of events likely to be associated with the drug)
- Rapidly increasing disproportionality* score
- Important public health impact (e.g. wide usage, number of cases, significant off-label use, direct-to-consumer programs)
- Easily retrievable data elements from database fields that are suggestive of a relationship with the drug (e.g. positive rechallenge, short time-to-onset, presence of literature cases in a case series)
- Temporal clustering of events

*   *triage algorithms implemented at WHO-UMC*

Impact analysis is therefore a systematic method of initial signal prioritization that provides guidance as to which signals should undergo a further more detailed evaluation.

(2) Further signal prioritization

Following initial signal triaging to determine which signals should undergo further evaluation a second prioritization step may be required in order to ensure that resources are appropriately allocated and that acceptable timelines are defined to meet public health and other obligations.

Table 10 summarizes points that may be considered in addition to those in Table 9 for further signal prioritization to establish how quickly detailed signal evaluation should be performed.

A mathematical pharmacovigilance issue prioritization tool has been developed and piloted at MHRA by Seabroke & Waller (publication in progress). The tool builds on the principles of impact analysis and includes other factors (such as those in Table 10) that may be important in determining acceptable timelines for signals requiring more detailed evaluation.

Table 10: Points to consider for further signal prioritization, not in hierarchical order (see 5, 6, 7)

- Reported/observed in a vulnerable population (e.g. paediatric, pregnant women, geriatric, psychiatric)
- Occurrence during the first few years post launch (i.e. "newer drug"*)
- Drug with a high media attention
- Risk perception by general population
- Reports from multiple countries
- More than one data source provides positive evidence of a hazard
- Political obligations (e.g. ministerial concern)

* *triage algorithms implemented at WHO-UMC*

b. Signal evaluation

Data/information quality and completeness are paramount to signal evaluation. As such, evaluating a signal requires a multi-faceted approach: (a) to collect the evidence to evaluate whether there is a causal link between the event and the administration of the medicinal product, (b) to determine whether the signal represents a potential or identified risk and, if this is the case, to characterize the qualitative and quantitative profile of the risk, and, (c) if a risk has been characterized, to communicate the risk and to propose measures aimed at preventing its occurrence or minimizing its consequences.

(1) Obtaining a consistent approach across all sources of safety data

The choice of a medically acceptable case definition, i.e. a set of terms consistent with the adverse event/disorder under evaluation, will be critical for searching for supportive information in all safety data sources. The challenge is to know when a symptom/sign constellation may represent a diagnosis of a potentially important medical condition. Accordingly, the set of terms that will be chosen may encompass a putative diagnosis of the condition under investigation with its main signs, symptoms, or complications (i.e. narrow search), or the search may expand to include less specific terms of related syndromes or less frequent signs, symptoms or complications (i.e. broad search) [for further details, please consult 10, 11, 12, 13]. In this respect, the inclusion of potential complications of the adverse effect in the case definition is important as they are key determinants of the level of risk.

As a general rule, the final signal evaluation report that serves to document a signal should include a reference in the "Material and Methods" section about the dictionary (usually MedDRA) used in the search strategies, the dictionary version and a description of all data sources that have been investigated.

(2) Assessing the strength of evidence from immediately available sources

It is not generally possible to specify exactly how and when a signal becomes a potential or identified risk. The presence and congruence of specific criteria (see Table 11) relating to the collective evidence help the confirmation process of when the index signal constitutes a risk. It is immediately obvious that the evaluation of a signal relies heavily on the clinical insight and pharmacological knowledge of the individual or the team performing the analysis. A team-based approach by a Safety Management Team (SMT) (14) generally provides the most comprehensive clinical and pharmaceutical experience necessary to guarantee the quality of a signal evaluation. The Safety Management Team (SMT) is a multi-disciplinary team which includes members from all relevant functions that are necessary to provide integrated assessments of safety data from multiple sources for a drug in the pre- or post-marketing phase.

Table 11: Criteria to be considered for evaluating a signal (modified from *1, 15, 16*)

Criteria to consider when reviewing a signal from a case series

- positive re-challenge(s) and/or de-challenge
- known mechanism (including class effect) or biological plausibility
- plausible and consistent time-to-onset between cases
- consistency between cases in the pattern of symptoms
- lack of confounding factors in the reported cases (particularly co-morbidities or co-medications)
- appropriate differential diagnoses are provided in the cases (e.g. literature reports) and concentrate on objective rather than subjective data
- putative signal occurs in younger age groups (e.g. children, infants and/or adolescents)
- signal observed in intentional or unintentional (e.g. drug-drug or drug-disease interactions) overdose situations
- existence of identifiable subgroups at particular risk
- positive dose response
- high frequency of reports (outside "stimulated" reporting)
- low natural background incidence of the putative signal in the treated population
- lack of alternative explanations

Criteria to consider when reviewing evidence from other sources

A. Clinical data (including pharmacodynamic, pharmacokinetic and interaction studies, primary or secondary pharmacology, dose-response, therapeutic explanatory and therapeutic confirmatory in well designed studies) (*17*)

- statistically significant difference (i.e. event [terms compatible with the signal under evaluation], lab or biomarkers of safety) in the treated group over placebo (particularly in randomized, double-blind controlled clinical studies)
- consistent outcome (i.e. event, lab or biomarker of safety) in a study specifically designed to investigate the association between a drug and an adverse reaction
- positive dose response
- pharmacokinetic evidence for an interaction (e.g. drug, food or disease)
- relative increase (e.g. relative risk > 2 in one or several comparative clinical studies
- consistent trend in studies (even when not statistically significant)
- converging evidence from observational post-marketing studies

B. Preclinical data in well designed studies

- similar findings in animals (in safety pharmacology or animal toxicology studies)
- positive *in vitro* or *ex vivo* tests

C. Product quality data

The signal from a case series is analyzed to identify trends and patterns that may provide a clue about a potential association with a given drug. Cases are grouped according to the type of event (e.g. diagnosis or signs or symptoms), patients' characteristics or demographics (e.g. age, ethnicity [or country of reporting], gender, co-morbidities, co-medications), disease (e.g. indication) or event characteristics (e.g. time to onset, severity). Factors such as the presence or absence of a temporal association, confounders, a high quality positive re-challenge as well as a judgment on the biological plausibility of a putative mechanism that could be attributed to the drug, determine the strength of evidence associated with a given signal. Drugs with the same active principle(s), or with slight variations in chemical formula, formulation (e.g. short-versus long-acting formulations), dosage or posology may account for differences in the strength of a signal. The SMT should consider whether other drugs with the same mode of action are associated with similar types of events.

The signal should be verified in other safety data sources which can include pharmaceutical toxicology or poison centre databases, pre-clinical (*in vitro*, *ex vivo* or *in vivo*) animal studies, clinical trials (e.g. experimental studies or specifically designed safety studies), epidemiological studies (prospective or retrospective, e.g. using medical claims or electronic patient record databases), all relevant literature and regulatory (e.g. FDA, WHO) databases. The data from all other relevant sources should be reviewed for congruence (i.e. strengthening) or inconsistency (i.e. weakening) with the original signal.

Understanding the distinct characteristics of safety data sources is critical prior to drawing any conclusions about whether the original signal is a potential or identified risk. Differences exist between databases, such as prospective versus retrospective data collection, sample size, report type (e.g. solicited versus unsolicited), time lag prior to entry into a database, presence or absence of consumer reports, presence of duplicate reports, and duration of observation. Duration of drug exposure is important when reviewing the available evidence; for instance, the absence of evidence in short duration clinical trials is not evidence of absence. This should be taken into account when looking at pooled data.

In addition, the data collection and structure may differ between investigational trials, or between investigational trials and observational studies (e.g. free or fixed visit schedule, interval between visits, presence of an adjudication or ascertainment process for events) as well as the diagnostic methods used (e.g. use of diagnostic tests versus clinical diagnosis, use of biomarkers or validated laboratory tests).

When the primary comprehensive evaluation of the signal does not permit the drawing of any reasonable conclusion as to the presence of a risk, consultation with independent experts should be considered. When necessary, the objective of discussing a signal between internal (e.g. drug safety board) or external experts (e.g. academia) is to seek opinions on whether the signal represents a potential or identified risk, determine acceptable levels of risk in a larger context and to help formulate an appropriate comprehensive course of action, including further risk assessment or risk minimization, as necessary.

c. Options analysis

When a reasonable level of suspicion of an association between an event and a drug has not been reached or when the level of risk has not been established, the safety physician or team in charge of a drug will need to elaborate a course of action including one or more options as appropriate.

Such options may include proposals that help to better characterize a signal or that aim at minimizing a medically important potential or identified risk for patients or populations at large. Risks should be evaluated in terms of their characteristics (e.g. potential for prevention, seriousness/severity, reversibility, public health consequence) and their frequency (i.e. likelihood of occurrence). Table 12 summarizes the activities that can be considered to confirm or better characterize a signal, and to report or communicate a risk.

Table 12: Potential characterization, reporting and communication activities (modified from *18*, *19*)

Characterization
- targeted clinical investigations (e.g. mechanistic safety studies)
- comparative observational studies (cross-sectional study/survey, case-control study, cohort study, epidemiological studies; retrospective or prospective)
- enhanced monitoring or follow-up techniques
- active surveillance schemes (sentinel sites, drug event monitoring, registries)
- large simple clinical trials
- consult internal or external experts

Reporting to regulatory authorities
- regulatory documents (e.g. Annual Safety Reports, Risk Management Plan, Periodic Safety Update Reports)

Communication to patients and prescribers
- product label (e.g. addition to label or labelling update)
- patient package insert/Medguides
- Dear Health Care Professional letter

(1) Potential risk

Signals that have not been verified may still be potential risks. Under these circumstances, additional activities may be required to characterize the potential risk (i.e. quantification of the risk in terms of severity and frequency). This can be done through the approaches summarized in Table 12, as appropriate. The speed and extent with which these additional steps will be undertaken are primarily related to the perceived medical and public health importance of the signal in relation to the drug benefit, a determination that very much requires expert judgment and cross-functional input.

The role of epidemiology in signal and risk management is significant. Epidemiological studies can serve two purposes, evaluating the strength of an association between a drug and a signal or estimating a risk in the population. Epidemiology can inform the determination of whether an association between the putative drug exposure and the outcome of interest is present, or can contribute to the quantification or population-level characteristics of a potential or identified risk. Epidemiology also provides context to the reports, observations, or signals, i.e. puts the event(s) in question into perspective by providing background rates of the event(s) in the population at risk that can be used as a point of reference. For instance, a single spontaneous report of a serious event would require some knowledge of the occurrence of this event in the appropriate population, with the understanding that reporting rates cannot be inferred to represent true incidence, even when adjusted for actual exposure or exposure surrogates (e.g. sales or distribution).

As alluded to earlier, not all signals will require an epidemiological follow-up study e.g. minor non-serious reactions. Those signals selected for further evaluation may necessitate such study depending on several factors, including, but not limited to, the following:

1. *The context*: the seriousness of the event and its potential impact on the benefit:risk balance of a product are key determinants to consider whether the additional confidence gained from an epidemiological study is justified in comparison to other actions. For example, a signal of thrombocytopenia following vaccination is clearly different from a similar signal following the taking of an oncology drug (i.e. further investigation would be required in the first instance, thrombocytopenia would be expected in the second).

2. *The feasibility*: the decision to undertake an epidemiological study is tempered by certain practical issues, such as availability of data and the frequency of the outcome of interest in the treated population as well as in the general population. If an adverse event is very rare, e.g. occurs between 1 in 100,000 and 1 in one million exposed persons, a prospective study would likely not be feasible, and few databases exist that could be used to study this event.

3. *The availability of suitable databases*, including the type and quality of data that would be required to adequately answer the relevant scientific questions

4. *The available resources*: no regulators, academics, or the pharmaceutical industry have infinite resources to investigate all signals generated by the mechanisms used by these different groups. Thus, the prioritization, as outlined in section a, is worth considering when deciding whether to initiate such studies. However, it is recognized that a certain amount of subjectivity will, of necessity, influence the final decision.

(2) Identified risk

Identified risks are those that emerge from verified signals. In other words, the index signal discussed in section b has been sufficiently well documented and confirmed by other available independent sources. The risk associated with that signal may or may not have been well quantified but there is general consensus that such a risk exists and is associated with the drug.

New identified risks warrant prompt actions which include such key steps as informing competent authorities, e.g. via updating the CSI and product labelling, and, if warranted, additional communications with patients and prescribers, e.g. via direct Dear Health Care Professional letter, RMP, PSUR, or other appropriate means based on local laws/regulations depending on the potential impact of the risk on the medicinal product's risk-benefit profile or to protect public health.

d. Reporting and communicating signals

Reporting is the spontaneous process, initiated by either a Marketing Authorization Holder (MAH) or a regulator, of informing each other on a signal/risk with a drug, while communicating is the process initiated by MAH or regulators to inform the public about a safety concern.

Reporting a signal is one of the most critical and sensitive matters of signal management. Expert judgment is inherent to the decisions about when a signal is sufficiently verified to be reported. As indicated earlier, approaches that could facilitate early discussions between a MAH and a regulator on whether the signal represents a potential or identified risk, determine acceptable levels of risk in a larger context and help formulate an appropriate comprehensive course of action are helpful. A pilot initiative has been undertaken to regularly and voluntarily report to the regulator all signals under evaluation by a MAH, irrespective of whether the signal information is still in the early stages or is only emerging (20).

Risk communication is the process of informing people about hazards to their health, encompassing the essential links between risk analysis, risk management, and informing the public. It is an exchange of information concerning the existence, nature, form, severity or acceptability of potential or identified health risks. Effective risk communication involves determining the types of information that interested and affected parties need and want, and presenting this information to them in a useful and meaningful way (21). Even though the communication process is particularly influenced by local laws/regulations, there have been sufficient agreements among experts to reach common ground on what and when to communicate. Communication experts generally agree that there are three main elements to focus on when communicating a potential or identified health risk: the message (i.e. short statements to inform and engage), the medium (i.e. multiple formats of information presentation aid comprehension) and the audience (e.g. general public, special interest groups, prescribers). The "Erice Declaration on Communicating Drug Safety Information" provides a set of guidances for an open, ethical, patient-centered communication that are easy to follow (22, 23, 24). Communicating drug safety information comprises objectives that are not mutually exclusive and should rather be considered as steps in a continuum: (a) communicating important emerging new signals that have not yet been fully analyzed or confirmed (see 19 and examples at 25), (b) communicating as a way to minimize safety risks (26, 27) and (c) communicating to support individual benefit:risk decisions.

Activities to communicate or to minimize a potential/identified risk fall outside the scope of this book and are discussed elsewhere in greater detail (but see also Chapter X).

e. Expectations for risk management planning

For any new drug, one of the aims of effective risk management planning is to identify risks from the gaps in the safety profile of the drug prior to registration/approval and plan for systematic collection of relevant data during the post-marketing phase. Risk management planning is also intended to address specific safety issues detected or suspected during the pre-marketing phase. Specific factors such as the extremes of age, pregnancy, impaired renal/hepatic function, other co-morbidities, extended duration of exposure, and clinical details of overdose or medication error are relevant. Important missing information is also within the scope of risk management.

In practice, it is likely that individual regulators will, for the most part, impose requirements on sponsors to address the issues through actions that are consistent with their global pharmacovigilance plans. Specific regional issues may need to be addressed through variations to the international risk management plans to meet local needs. It is possible that regulatory agencies may have well-founded legitimate reasons to require additional monitoring or an ongoing clinical study e.g. to investigate genetic polymorphism in a particular ethnic population. That being the case, it follows that other regulatory agencies should have the right to be appraised of any ongoing studies and of the requirements and timeframe involved in any additional monitoring program.

Currently, the EMA routinely requires the submission of a risk management plan with certain marketing authorization applications, and has published a template for the content required for these submissions (28). The United States has passed legislation called the Food and Drug Administration Amendments Act of 2007; Title IX of this act increases the agency's authority to manage the safety of marketed drugs. The legislation stipulates that manufacturers should provide the agency with risk evaluation and management strategies if there is a concern about the benefit-risk profile of the product. Such strategies include communication plans, patient registries, restricted distribution, etc. (29).

Individual companies have taken diverse approaches to risk management planning. Some organizations begin a formal process, including risk management plans and safety milestone assessments at pre-clinical development stages, while others begin this process in Phase III or peri-approval stages. The putative benefits of starting this risk management process in pre-clinical development include a safety-focused, proactive planning process at the start of development. However, given the limited knowledge that exists on compounds at these early stages, and the high attrition rate of compounds in Phase I and II, there may be limited value in formalized risk management activities for early development compounds. As the concept of formal benefit risk management planning across an entire portfolio is relatively new, further guidance from regulators may well be required to define the scope of necessary risk management planning.

Interested readers are referred to the relevant literature for further details on managing risks and developing a risk management plan (see 28, 29, 30, 31).

f. Conclusions and recommendations

Signal management is a process that requires a high-level standard operating procedure (SOP) describing:

- How signal prioritization and evaluation are approached (e.g. what does the signal prioritization imply? How are the sources of safety data queried? Who does the signal evaluation?);

- How risk determination is performed (e.g. what criteria have been considered and what data are available to qualify the risks?);

- How the best course of action is determined;

- When, how and to whom will the potential or identified risks be communicated.

Once a signal has been identified, the following activities should be undertaken:

- Triaging or evaluating for public health impact;

- Assessing the validity and strength of the index signal and identifying gaps that prevent understanding a potential association and whether the signal represents a potential or identified risk;

- Determining an appropriate case definition for searching all relevant safety data sources keeping in mind the limitations of each data source;

- Reviewing and compiling safety data in an overall assessment document;

- Analyzing the degree of congruence of safety data from other sources with the data from the original signal;

- Assessing the characteristics (e.g. potential for prevention, seriousness/ severity, reversibility, clinical or public health consequences) and the frequency (likelihood of occurrence) of the potential or identified risk associated with the signal;

- Identifying a proportionate course of action that includes the relevant activities necessary for further evaluation, communication and risk minimization, as appropriate.

References

1. Identifying and describing safety signals: from case reports to case series. In *Guidance for Industry – Good Pharmacovigilance Practices and Pharmacoepidemiologic Assessment.* Rockville, MD, FDA/CDER, 2005:4-12 (available at http://www.fda.gov/cder/guidance/6359OCC.pdf, accessed 26 November 2008).

2. Meyboom RHB et al. Signal selection and follow-up in pharmacovigilance. *Drug Safety*, 2002, 459-65.

3. Yee CL et al. Practical considerations in developing an automated signalling program within a pharmacovigilance department. *Drug Information Journal*, 2004, 38:293-300.

4. Bright RA, Nelson RC. Automated support for pharmacovigilance: a proposed system. *Pharmacoepidemiology and Drug Safety*, 2002, 11:121-5.

5. Ståhl M et al. Introducing triage logic as a new strategy for the detection of signals in the WHO Drug Monitoring Database. *Pharmacoepidemiology and Drug Safety*, 2004, 13:355-63.

6. Lindquist M. Use of triage strategies in the WHO signal-detection process. *Drug Safety*, 2007, 30:635-7.

7. van Puijenbroek EP et al. Determinants of signal detection in a spontaneous reporting system for adverse drug reactions. *British Journal of Clinical Pharmacology,* 2001, 52:579-86.

8. Waller PC, Heeley E, Moseley J. Impact analysis of signals detected from spontaneous adverse drug reaction reporting data. *Drug Safety*, 2005, 28:843-50.

9. Heeley E, Waller PC, Moseley J. Testing and implementing signal impact analysis in a regulatory setting – results of a pilot study. *Drug Safety*, 2005, 28:901-6.

10. Bankowski Z et al., eds. *Reporting adverse drug reactions – definitions of terms and criteria for their use.* Geneva, CIOMS, 1999.

11. ICH-endorsed guide for MedDRA users, MedDRA term selection: points to consider. ICH, 2008 (http://www.ich.org/MediaServer.jser?@_ID=4826&@_MODE=GLB, accessed 26 November 2008).

12. ICH-endorsed guide for MedDRA users on data output, MedDRA data retrieval and presentation: points to consider. ICH, 2008 (available at http://www.ich.org/MediaServer.jser?@_ID=4822&@_MODE=GLB, accessed 26 November 2008).

13. Definitions and Guidelines. In *The Brighton Collaboration – Setting Standards in Vaccine Safety* (www.brightoncollaboration.org, accessed 26 November 2008).

14. Good pharmacovigilance and risk management practices: systematic approach to managing safety during clinical development. In *Management of Safety Information from Clinical Trials – Report of CIOMS Working Group VI.* Geneva, CIOMS, 2005:58-59.

15. Table 1. In *Guidelines for preparing core clinical-safety information on drugs – Report of CIOMS Working Group III.* Geneva, CIOMS, 1995:46-47.

16. Bradford Hill A. The environment and disease: association or causation. *Proc R Soc Med,* 1965, 58:295-330.

17. ICH – General considerations for clinical trials E8. ICH, 1997.

18. Annex – Pharmacovigilance methods in *ICH E2E Pharmacovigilance Planning* (http://www.ich.org/cache/compo/276-254-1.html, accessed 26 November 2008).

19. Guidance – Drug Safety Information – FDA's Communication to the Public. Rockville, MD, FDA/CDER, 2007 (http://www.fda.gov/Cder/guidance/7477fnl.pdf, accessed 26 November 2008).

20. Swain E et al. Early communication of drug safety concerns. *Pharmacoepidemiology and Drug Safety*, 2010, 19: 232-237.

21. Health Canada, Decision-making framework for identifying, assessing and managing health risks, 1 August 2000 (http://www.hc-sc.gc.ca/ahc-asc/pubs/hpfb-dgpsa/risk-risques_cp-pc_e. html, accessed 26 November 2008).

22. Hugman B. The Erice declaration – the critical role of communication in drug safety. *Drug Safety*, 2006, 29:91-3.

23. The Uppsala Monitoring Centre. *Effective communications in pharmacovigilance, the Erice report.* Uppsala, WHO/UMC, 1998.

24. Appendix 1: The Erice declaration on communicating drug safety information. In *Current Challenges in Pharmacovigilance: Report of CIOMS Working Group V.* Geneva, CIOMS, 2001:219-200.

25. FDA Drug Safety Newsletter (http://www.fda.gov/CDER/dsn/factsheet.htm, accessed 26 November 2008).

26. Template for rapid alert in pharmacovigilance. In *Volume 9A of the Rules Governing Medicinal Products in the European Union – Guidelines on Pharmacovigilance for medicinal products for Human Use.* EMEA, 2007, 214-215.

27. Template for non-urgent information in pharmacovigilance. In *Volume 9A of the Rules Governing Medicinal Products in the European Union – Guidelines on Pharmacovigilance for medicinal products for Human Use*. EMEA, 2007: 216-217.

28. Annex C: Template for EU risk management plan (EU-RMP) (http://eudravigilance.emea.europa.eu/human/docs/19263206en.pdf, accessed 26 November 2008, and http://eudravigilance.emea.europa.eu/human/EURiskManagementPlans.asp accessed 26 November 2008).

29. Risk evaluation and mitigation strategies. In *One Hundred Tenth Congress of the United States of America*, Title IX, HR 3580, Sec 505-1:105-16 (http://www.fda.gov/oc/initiatives/HR3580.pdf, accessed 26 November 2008).

30. *Guidance for Industry – development and use of risk minimization action plans*. FDA, 2005 (http://www.fda.gov/cder/Guidance/6358fnl.pdf, accessed 26 November 2008).

31. Requirements for risk management systems. In *Volume 9A of the Rules Governing Medicinal Products in the European Union – Guidelines on Pharmacovigilance for medicinal products for Human Use*. EMEA, 2007:34-53 (http://ec.europa.eu/enterprise/pharmaceuticals/eudralex/vol-9/pdf/vol9_2007-07_upd07.pdf, accessed 26 November 2008).

X

Future directions in signal detection, evaluation and communication

a. Wider considerations

With the advent of the 21st century, the field of pharmacovigilance is poised to enter an exciting new era. Major changes are afoot, changes that reflect a growing recognition that pharmacovigilance is a global endeavor that must employ state-of-the-art methods and draw upon the best quality evidence if it is to be effective in protecting the public's health and safety. A number of external forces have been instrumental in instigating this transformation, in particular the increasing demand by regulators for formal benefit/risk assessments as part of the risk minimization strategy development process for a new product. However, in addition to risk identification and prioritization, pharmacovigilance data are also potentially useful for evaluating the effectiveness of interventions designed to minimize identified risks.

The goal of the CIOMS VIII Report is to set forth strategic recommendations for managing the "lifecycle" of a drug safety signal identified in spontaneous reporting systems (SRS). The key phases in the drug safety signal lifecycle were identified as being signal detection, signal prioritization, signal evaluation, and, in cases where an actual risk was identified, appropriate communication and implementation of risk minimization efforts. Strategic recommendations corresponding to the conduct of signal detection, prioritization and evaluation have been set forth in prior chapters of this document. The purpose of this final chapter is to highlight important future directions in pharmacovigilance pertaining to signal detection, evaluation and risk management interventions, and to discuss approaches to communicating signal information.

b. New directions in data mining algorithms (DMAs)

(1) Sensitivity and specificity

Data mining in pharmacovigilance is a dynamic field. To date, a number of data mining algorithms (DMAs) or data mining "tools" have been developed and applied to different SRS. These include the WHO database, the United States FDA's AERS database, EMA's EudraVigilance database, and internal pharmaceutical company databases. Determination of which of these DMAs is most appropriate for signal detection in SRS, however, has yet to be made. While in clinical medicine, a new tool or test typically undergoes extensive analysis for sensitivity, specificity and positive predictive value, there has been limited work of this type in terms of DMAs. For any data mining tool, a thorough evaluation of signal threshold criteria should be conducted, as well as an analysis of the impact that a higher or lower threshold has on the sensitivity, specificity and predictive value of the algorithm. This type of formal assessment needs to be undertaken before optimum algorithms for SRS can be identified in any particular setting.

(2) Denominators

A fundamental limitation of all SRS is the lack of a denominator. Patient-level drug usage data has been proposed as one possible denominator candidate, and researchers at the FDA and the WHO-UMC have been using commercial sales estimates or number of prescriptions dispensed to estimate reporting rates (1, 2). Another denominator that has been used is an estimated "number of patients exposed to a given drug". This estimate is based on extrapolation from volume of manufactured active ingredient available. A fourth denominator candidate is the "number of unique individuals dispensed the drug." This estimate is derived from prescription drug data that permits, through the use of a proprietary algorithm, identification of unique patients who have filled a prescription for the drug at a retail pharmacy (3).

(3) Screening for drug-drug interactions

The potential usefulness of SRS databases for routine drug-drug interaction (DDI) screening has been explored intensively in recent years and several new methods have been developed. These include simple frequentist approaches, as well as more complex Bayesian methods such as Lasso Logistic Regression (4). In some scenarios, however, simpler methods may be more effective and should not be overlooked (5).

While research into the optimal statistical method for DDI screening is ongoing, routine screening for DDIs may ultimately become a standard component of automated signal detection activities in SRS databases (6). The WHO-UMC has developed methodology to partially automate interaction searches (7), and is conducting further work on routine interaction screening.

(4) Confirmatory data analysis

Can data mining of a SRS be used to confirm a previously identified signal? The classic methods of clinical evaluation are widely used to assess the evidence for a causal relationship based on Bradford Hill criteria. While additional data mining may provide further information, it cannot supplant the role of clinical evaluation. For confirmation of a signal, a non-SRS dataset is likely to be most informative.

The detection of new aspects of known ADRs is an important element of drug safety surveillance; but has received relatively little attention in the data mining literature, and has yet to be fully explored. The limited available research suggests that 2x2 based methods may be useful for detecting changes in known ADRs. In principle, multivariate techniques or pattern recognition have the potential to further elucidate such phenomena.

Potential future enhancements of data mining in SRS datasets will require incorporating other data elements into existing algorithms, such as adverse event onset interval, positive re-challenge/de-challenge, product lot information, and reporter type.

c. Data mining in non-SRS datasets

A number of other databases can be used to detect signals using data mining techniques. The main advantage of these data sources is that there is a well defined patient denominator from which drug-event pairs are arising, thereby permitting the calculation of incidence rates and comparisons of incidence rates between different drugs or different patient subgroups.

(1) Computerized longitudinal healthcare databases

Computerized databases containing health care information, including electronic medical records databases and medical claims databases, have been used extensively to evaluate previously identified signals in formal, protocol-driven, epidemiological studies targeted at specific safety questions, using longitudinal cohort or case-control analytical methods. Since 2004, data mining of longitudinal healthcare claims records has been conducted at the WHO-UMC (8). In addition, several large United States healthcare databases, such as the Veteran Affairs and Medicare databases, are now also being used for data mining purposes. Also, various commercial vendors of automated healthcare databases are offering signal detection tools for application to computerized healthcare databases. Despite this trend, however, the use of large health care claims or electronic medical record data for signal detection is still in its infancy. One vital and as yet unaddressed question is whether data mining of these large health care databases for signal detection yields a higher positive predictive value than data mining of SRS datasets.

Several different techniques have been developed for data mining in large health care databases. These include sequential monitoring methods, retrospective screening, continuous disproportionality screening, and meta-analysis.

(2) Sequential monitoring

Sequential monitoring, or rapid cycle analysis, involves close-to-real-time prospective monitoring for pre-specified events of special interest or concern (also referred to as Designated Medical Events (DMEs) and Targeted Medical Events (TMEs)). With this approach, rates of adverse events are rapidly assessed during the early period of drug marketing post-licensure.

A retrospective proof-of-concept study of such an approach was conducted by Davis et al. for the Vaccine Safety Datalink project in the United States (9). Using Sequential Probability Ratio Testing (SPRT) methodology, the authors showed that a number of confirmed safety signals would have been detected in managed care data prior to their detection using SRS data.

The limitations of this approach, similar to conventional observational studies, however, are issues related to bias (e.g. channeling bias, confounding by severity). Another limitation is the need to define an *a priori* list of events to be used for monitoring purposes when it is not always clear in advance which and how many such events to include. Additionally, once a signal is detected, it requires evaluation, an exercise best conducted in a separate database. If use of a separate database is not feasible, however, the existing dataset can be randomly divided into test and validation subsets. This approach, however, sacrifices some degree of sensitivity in detecting signals.

Sequential monitoring also requires timely access to updated patient data. For the implementation of practical rapid cycle analyses of newly licensed medicinal products, close collaboration between users of active surveillance systems (e.g. regulators, drug manufacturers, clinicians, pharmacists, etc.) and patient data vendors is needed. Not least, development of such a system requires the investment of substantial resources.

(3) Cross-sectional screening or data mining

Retrospective periodic screening of patient health record databases for unusual epidemiological patterns/drug-event associations is another approach for signal detection. This activity is akin to data mining for signals in SRS databases, except that instead of calculating relative reporting rate ratios (such as PRR, ROR, EBGM, IC, etc.), event incidence [density] rate ratios are determined for a large list of drug-event pairs.

(4) Continuous disproportionality screening

Continuous disproportionality screening involves ongoing evaluation of the disproportionality of events for patients using the unexposed period for control. The method has the advantages of being suitable for continuous monitoring and visualization of trends in events but may lack generalizability to other data sets in its current form. Bate et al. retrospectively evaluated the use of continuous disproportionality screening in a primary care records database in the United Kingdom and concluded that data mining in longitudinal healthcare datasets can identify known signals, as well as new plausible signals, though the predictive value needs further evaluation (10). The WHO-UMC is introducing the method more widely for signal detection in longitudinal databases in other countries. The method has the advantage of finding signals early, with two types of control, but suffers from the problems of multiple analysis, and limitations in the records and terminology. A major advantage is the availability of a transparent, chronological record of the disproportionalities in the exposed cohort compared with controls over time. Moreover, since the method can detect disproportionalities between positive as well as negative events before and after treatment, it might have value in benefit-risk studies.

(5) Data mining, meta-analysis and clinical trial datasets

Disproportionality analysis relies on the dichotomous classification of suspect drugs and associated events. In a sense, this involves collapsing a great deal of information on multiple drugs and events into two basic categories. This potential loss of information has stimulated research into multivariate methods. Meta-analyses of pooled individual data across multiple trials are increasingly being done, and have resulted in several safety signals being detected or confirmed. Thus, pooled or meta-analyses of clinical trial datasets should be considered integral components of a pharmacovigilance system in the post-marketing as well as the pre-marketing period.

d. Use of ICSRs to evaluate impact of risk minimization

ICSR data can potentially be used to evaluate the impact of risk minimization interventions. It can be used to evaluate a variety of different types of interventions using a basic pre-post design with an appropriate comparator arm. This is a potentially useful application that deserves further research attention.

e. Communication of signal information

Signal communication represents a key step in the signal detection and evaluation process. From a public health perspective, timely and effective communication of signal information to relevant stakeholders is the linchpin upon which effective pharmacovigilance practice rests. Growing appreciation of the vital role risk communication has to play in drug safety is evident in a number of recent governmental projects, including the FDA's regular publication initiative, and MHRA's Patient Information Expert Advisory Group. Although certain principles of risk communication have been recognized as important, no consensus has yet emerged in regard to best practices. Communication of signal information involves some unique challenges. Such challenges include development and delivery of appropriate messages, and timing of information release to key stakeholder groups.

(1) Message content and delivery

Effective communication regarding an emerging drug safety risk should involve, at minimum, a description of the potential safety issue, the data (sometimes preliminary) which generated it, additional data that is currently being or will be reviewed, and an approximate time frame for the ongoing safety review to be completed. Both the content and framing of the signal information however, require tailoring for each of the key stakeholder groups involved: healthcare professionals/prescribers, patients, their caregivers, and the general public. Development of message content should be guided by evidence-based research on adult learning, and human cognition. Important additional considerations for patients include sensitivity to differences in culture, language of origin, and health literacy level.

Although labeling materials represent the foundation for the provision of drug safety information, revisions to labeling take time and hence cannot be utilized for the purposes of rapidly conveying new signal information to healthcare providers and patients. For time-sensitive communications, a variety of communication modalities should be employed, including print and electronic media as well as broadcast public service announcements. Another rapid safety communication method that can be employed is the posting of signals on designated web sites. The FDA has begun using such an approach. Each quarter, it posts a list of drugs deemed to have a potential safety signal on the Consumer Health information page of its web site, as well as on WebMD.com, a health information web site (11). The drugs posted on these sites have had one or more serious potential risks or new safety information reported to AERS in the previous three months. The appearance of a drug on this list does not mean that the FDA has concluded that the drug has this listed risk. Instead, it means that the FDA has identified a potential safety issue that it is evaluating, but has not as yet identified a cause and effect relationship (*12*). Research is being undertaken on the value of the FDA signal publication.

(2)   Timing of signal communication

A signal is only an indicator of a potential safety problem. Further evaluation is required before it can be definitively determined to be an actual risk. Such an evaluation requires time as it involves data review. The timing of signal communication can be conducted in stages that correspond with this signal evaluation process. The initial release of information can assume the form of an alert or "early communication" about the newly detected signal. Subsequent communications can follow as "safety updates" that are intended to impart new information gained through review of one or more sources of additional data. Once sufficient data have been reviewed to permit risk determination with reasonable certitude, separate communications for 1) healthcare professionals/prescribers, and 2) to patients and caregivers, should be developed and distributed. Such communications can take the form of information sheets (for healthcare professionals) and/or Public Health Advisories or equivalent (for patients and caregivers).

Once available data have been fully analyzed, additional communication may occur before any regulatory action is taken especially in the following circumstances:

- If communicating information about the safety issue could change the risk/benefit profile for the drug which may, in turn, affect decisions about prescribing or using the drug;
- When there are specific actions that may be taken by healthcare professionals or patients to prevent harm which can include preventing medication errors;
- If the safety issue involves an unapproved use and the use of the medicine poses a risk of harm;
- If the safety issue affects a vulnerable population.

f.   Conclusions and recommendations

- Assessing the sensitivity and specificity of DMAs is essential for further development and application of these tools.
- The feasibility and analytic impact of employing alternative types of denominator candidates in SRS data requires evaluation.
- Consideration should be given to using multiple data sets as part of the signal evaluation process.
- There is a need for further research to determine whether data mining of healthcare administrative claims databases for signal detection yields a higher positive predictive value than data mining of SRS datasets.
- Given the importance of clinical trials as sources of signals in the post-marketing period, pooled or meta-analyses of clinical trial datasets should be considered integral components of a pharmacovigilance system.

- Signal communication may benefit from using a 'staged' approach, one that corresponds to the different phases of the signal detection and evaluation process.

- Communication of signal information should be guided by the latest evidence regarding adult learning and human cognition, and consideration should be given to tailoring content for specific stakeholder audiences.

- Further research needs to be conducted to determine when, what, and how signal information should be communicated most effectively. In particular, a range of communication modalities needs to be considered and evaluated, including newly emerging communication technologies as well as more established methods.

In the past, CIOMS has used a variety of means for disseminating its deliberations, particularly to those outside the WHO Program. For many pharmacovigilance topics CIOMS has addressed to date, 'harmonization' (i.e. sharing, understanding and cooperating) as opposed to 'standardization' (regulations identifying a set of fixed approaches or methods that must be used) has often been advocated. Such is the case in regard to signal detection and signal management activities, including data mining methodologies. Unanimously, the Working Group agreed that fixed or regulated standards would not be appropriate at this, or potentially any, juncture. By definition, signal detection and management activities require individualized approaches and lateral thinking. Data mining is one tool in this regard and its full potential, both for benefit and misuse, has yet to be fully realized.

References

1. Szarfman A, Machado SG, O'Neill RT. Use of screening algorithms and computer systems to efficiently signal higher-than-expected combinations of drugs and events in the US FDA's spontaneous reports database. *Drug Safety*, 2002, 25:381-392.

2. Lindquist M et al. How does cystitis affect a comparative risk profile of tiaprofenic acid with other non-steroidal anti-inflammatory drugs? An international study based on spontaneous reports and drug usage data. ADR Signals Analysis Project (ASAP) Team. *Pharmacol Toxicol,* 1997, 80(5):211-7.

3. Smith MY et al. Quantifying morbidity associated with the abuse and misuse of opioid analgesics: a comparison of two approaches. *Clinical Toxicology*, 2007, 45(1):23-30.

4. Caster O et al. Large scale regression-based pattern discovery: the example of screening in the WHO Global Drug Safety database. (http://www.stat.columbia.edu/~madigan/PAPERS/sam-2.pdf, accessed 18 December 2009)

5. Lindquist M et al. New pharmacovigilance information on an old drug – an international study of spontaneous reports on Digoxin. *Drug Investigation*, 1994, 8:73-80.

6. Strandell J et al. Drug-drug interactions – a preventable patient safety issue? *British Journal of Clinical Pharmacology,* 2008, 65(1):144-146.

7. Norén GN et al. A statistical methodology for drug-drug interaction surveillance. *Statistics in Medicine*, 2008. 27(16):3057-70.

8. Norén GN et al. Temporal pattern discovery for trends and transient effects: its application to patient records. In ACM *SIGKDD International Conference on Knowledge Discovery and Data Mining*, 2008, Las Vegas, Nevada, USA: KDD '08. ACM.

9. Davis RL et al. Active surveillance of vaccine safety: a system to detect early signs of adverse events. *Epidemiology*, 2005, 16(3):336-341

10. Bate A et al. Knowledge finding in IMS disease analyser Mediplus UK database – effective data mining in longitudinal patient safety data. Drug Safety, 2004, 27:917-918.

11. Houghton M. FDA partners with WebMD for broader dissemination of product safety info. FDC Reports: Health News Daily – 4 December 2008. Direct URL to article: http://thegraysheet. elsevierbi.com/cs/Satellite?c=Page&cid=1216099165884&pagename=FDCReports/Page/Pag eNavigatorWrapper&autoLogin=yes&queryStr=resultpage*ArticleDetail:ArticleDetailWrapp er/pii*081204g1/pubdate*20081204/qbax*0aJ842L2KIdp7ttotwzI5w==&jid=gray&pii=0812 04g1&pubdate=20081204# Accessed online at The Pink Sheet Daily on 17 December 2009: http://thepinksheetdaily.elsevierbi.com/cs/Satellite?c=Page&cid=1216099237581&pagename= pdly/Page/MarketingWrapper&rendermode=previewnoinsite>

12. Personal communication, G. Dal Pan, 30 November 2008.

Glossary and acronyms

Active surveillance

An active surveillance system has been defined by the World Health Organization as the collection of case safety information as a continuous pre-organized process.

The Importance of Pharmacovigilance: Safety Monitoring of Medicinal Products. Geneva, WHO, 2002.

Active surveillance can be (1) drug based: identifying adverse events in patients taking certain products, (2) setting based: identifying adverse events in certain health care settings where they are likely to present for treatment (e.g. emergency departments, etc.), or (3) event based: identifying adverse events that are likely to be associated with medical products (e.g. acute liver failure).

Guidance for Industry: Good Pharmacovgilance Practices and Pharmacoepidemiology Assessment. Rockville, MD, Food and Drug Administration (FDA), March 2005. (http://www.fda.gov/downloads/RegulatoryInformation/Guidances/UCM126834.pdf, accessed 11 December 2009).

Adverse drug reaction (ADR)

A noxious and unintended response to a medicinal product for which there is a reasonable possibility that the product caused the response. The phrase "response to a medicinal product" means that a causal relationship between a medicinal product and an adverse event is at least a reasonable possibility. The phrase "a reasonable possibility" means that there are facts, evidence, or arguments to support a causal association with the medicinal product.

ICH E2A Guideline for Industry: Clinical Safety Data Management: Definitions and Standards for Expedited Reporting. Step 5 as of October 1994. (http://www.ich.org/LOB/media/MEDIA436.pdf, accessed 11 December 2009).

Note: From a regulatory perspective, all spontaneous reports are considered "suspected" ADRs in that they convey the suspicions of the reporters. A causality assessment by the regulatory authority may indicate whether there could be alternative explanations for the observed adverse event other than the suspect drug. It should be noted that although overdose is not included in the basic definition of an adverse drug reaction in the post-approval environment, information regarding overdose, abuse and misuse should be included as part of the risk assessment of any medicinal product.

Adverse event (AE)

Any untoward medical occurrence in a patient or clinical investigation subject administered a pharmaceutical product which does not necessarily have a causal relationship with this treatment.

Note: An adverse event can therefore be any unfavourable and unintended sign (including an abnormal laboratory finding), symptom, or disease temporally associated with the use of a medicinal (investigational) product, whether or not related to the medicinal (investigational) product.

Guideline for Good Clinical Practice, ICH Harmonised Tripartite Guideline, E6(R1), Curren*t Step 4 version,* dated 10 June 2006 *(including Post Step 4 corrections).* (http://www.ich.org/LOB/media/MEDIA482.pdf, accessed 11 December 2009).

Alert

An identified risk associated with the use of medicinal products which requires urgent measures to protect patients.

Bayesian Confidence Propagation Neural Network (BCPNN)

Empirical Bayesian algorithm used for signal detection in spontaneous report databases.

Causality assessment

The evaluation of the likelihood that a medicine was the causative agent of an observed adverse event in a specific individual. Causality assessment is usually made according to established algorithms.

Adapted from: *Glossary of terms used in Pharmacovigilance.* WHO Collaborating Centre for International Drug Monitoring, Uppsala. (http://www.who-umc.org/graphics/8321.pdf, accessed 11 December 2009).

Cohort event monitoring (CEM)

A surveillance method that requests prescribers to report all observed adverse events, regardless of whether or not they are suspected adverse drug reactions, for identified patients receiving a specific drug. Also called prescription event monitoring.

Glossary of terms used in Pharmacovigilance. WHO Collaborating Centre for International Drug Monitoring, Uppsala. (http://www.who-umc.org/graphics/8321. pdf, accessed 11 December 2009).

Data mining

Any computational method used to automatically extract useful information from a large amount of data. Data mining is a form of exploratory data analysis.

Adapted from: Hand, Manilla and Smyth. *Principles of data mining*. Cambridge, MA, USA. MIT Press, 2001.

Designated medical event (DME)

Adverse events considered rare, serious, and associated with a high drug-attributable risk and which constitute an alarm with as few as one to three reports. Examples include Stevens-Johnson syndrome, toxic epidermal necrolysis, hepatic failure, anaphylaxis, aplastic anaemia and torsade de pointes.

Hauben M et al. The role of data mining in pharmacovigilance. *Expert Opinion in Drug Safety*, 2005, 4:929-948.

Disproportionality analysis/Analysis of disproportionate reporting

The application of computer-assisted computational and statistical methods to large safety databases for the purpose of systematically identifying drug-event pairs reported at disproportionately higher frequencies relative to what a statistical independence model would predict.

Almenoff J et al. Perspectives on the use of data mining in pharmacovigilance. *Drug Safety*, 2005, 28:981-1007.

Drug-event pair

A combination of a medicinal product and an adverse event which has appeared in at least one case report entered in a spontaneous report database.

Frequentist statistics

Probabilities viewed as a long term frequency with an assumption of a repeatable experiment or sampling mechanism.

Hazard

A situation that under particular circumstances could lead to harm. A source of danger.

Benefit-Risk Balance for Marketed Drugs: Evaluating Safety Signals. Report of CIOMS Working Group IV. Geneva, CIOMS, 1998.

Identified risk

An untoward occurrence for which there is adequate evidence of an association with the medicinal product of interest.

Guideline on Risk Management Systems for medicinal products for human use, Vol 9A of Eudralex, Chapter I.3, March 2007. (http://ec.europa.eu/enterprise/pharmaceuticals/eudralex/vol-9/pdf/vol9_2007-07_upd07.pdf, accessed 11 December 2009).

Multi-Item Gamma Poisson Shrinkage (MGPS)

Empirical Bayesian algorithm used for signal detection in spontaneous report databases.

Passive surveillance (of spontaneous reports)

A surveillance method that relies on healthcare providers (and consumers in some countries) to take the initiative in communicating suspicions of adverse drug reactions that may have occurred in individual patients to a spontaneous reporting system.

Pharmacoepidemiology

Study of the use and effects of drugs in large populations.

Glossary of terms used in Pharmacovigilance. WHO Collaborating Centre for International Drug Monitoring, Uppsala. (http://www.who-umc.org/graphics/8321. pdf, accessed 11 December 2009).

Pharmacovigilance

The science and activities relating to the detection, assessment, understanding and prevention of adverse effects or any other drug-related problem.

Glossary of terms used in Pharmacovigilance. WHO Collaborating Centre for International Drug Monitoring, Uppsala. (http://www.who-umc.org/graphics/8321. pdf, accessed 11 December 2009).

Post-authorization

The stage in the life-cycle of a medicinal product that follows the granting of the marketing authorization, after which the product may be placed on the market.

Post-marketing

The stage when a drug is available on the market.

Glossary of terms used in Pharmacovigilance. WHO Collaborating Centre for International Drug Monitoring, Uppsala. (http://www.who-umc.org/graphics/8321. pdf, accessed 11 December 2009).

Post-marketing surveillance

Monitoring for adverse reactions to marketed products.

Adapted from Glossary of MHRA terms. (http://www.mhra.gov.uk/home/ idcplg?IdcService=SS_GET_PAGE&nodeId=408, accessed 11 December 2009).

Potential risk

An untoward occurrence for which there is some basis for suspicion of an association with the medicinal product of interest but where this association has not been confirmed.

Guideline on Risk Management Systems for medicinal products for human use, Vol 9A of Eudralex, Chapter I.3, March 2007. (http://ec.europa.eu/enterprise/pharmaceuticals/eudralex/vol-9/pdf/vol9_2007-07_upd07.pdf, accessed 11 December 2009).

Pre-authorization

The stage in the life-cycle of a medicinal product before the drug has obtained a marketing authorization.

Note: A marketing authorization pertains to each indication. Once authorized for one indication, a drug still may be in pre-authorization development for another indication.

ICH Topic E8. General Considerations for Clinical Trials. 17 July 1997. (http://www.ich.org/LOB/media/MEDIA484.pdf, accessed 11 December 2009).

Pre-marketing

The stage before a drug is available for prescription or sale to the public. Usually synonymous with pre-approval or pre-authorization.

Adapted from *Glossary of terms used in Pharmacovigilance,* WHO Collaborating Centre for International Drug Monitoring, Uppsala. (http://www.who-umc.org/graphics/8321.pdf, accessed 11 December 2009).

Prescription event monitoring (PEM) or Cohort event monitoring (CEM)

A surveillance method that requests prescribers to report all observed adverse events, regardless of whether or not they are suspected adverse drug reactions, for identified patients receiving a specific drug. Also more accurately named "cohort-event monitoring".

Glossary of terms used in Pharmacovigilance. WHO Collaborating Centre for International Drug Monitoring, Uppsala. (http://www.who-umc.org/graphics/8321.pdf, accessed 11 December 2009).

Proportional reporting ratio (PRR)

The proportion of reports for an event that involve a particular drug compared to the proportion of reports of this event for all drugs in a spontaneous report database. This is expressed as a ratio and reflects the observed/expected values for that event in the database.

Adapted from: Evans SJW et al. Use of proportional reporting ratios (PRRs) for signal generation from spontaneous adverse drug reaction reports. *Pharmacoepidemiology and Drug Safety* 2001, 10:483-486.

Qualitative signal detection

Case-by-case manual screening of each individual case report of a suspected adverse drug reaction submitted to a spontaneous reporting system that must be performed by an assessor. The assessor uses his/her human intellect to evaluate the likelihood that the adverse event was caused by the suspect drug.

Adapted from: Egberts TCG. Signal Detection: Historical Background. *Drug Safety* 2007, 30:607-609.

Quantitative signal detection

Refers to computational or statistical methods used to identify drug-event pairs (or higher-order combinations of drugs and events) that occur with disproportionately high frequency in large spontaneous report databases.

Almenoff J et al. Perspectives on the use of data mining in pharmacovigilance. *Drug Safety,* 2005, 28:981-1007.

Reporting odds ratio (ROR)

The odds (probability/1-probability) of finding an adverse event term among all case reports that mention a particular drug divided by the odds of finding the same adverse event term among all other case reports in the spontaneous report database that do not mention this drug.

Risk

The probability of developing an outcome.

Note: The term *risk* normally, but not always, refers to a negative outcome. When used for medicinal products, the concept of risk concerns adverse drug reactions. Contrary to *harm*, the concept of risk does not involve severity of an outcome. The time interval at risk should be specified.

Adapted from: Lindquist, M. The need for definitions in pharmacovigilance. *Drug Safety,* 2007, 30:825-830.

Risk assessment

Risk assessment consists of identifying and characterizing the nature, frequency, and severity of the risk associated with the use of a product. Risk assessment occurs throughout a product's lifecycle, from the early identification of a potential product, through the pre-marketing development process, and after approval during marketing.

FDA Guidance for Industry. Premarketing Risk Assessment. March 2005. (http://www.fda.gov/downloads/Drugs/GuidanceComplianceRegulatoryInformation/Guidances/ucm072002.pdf, accessed 11 December 2009).

Note: Risk assessment can be subdivided into risk estimation and risk evaluation.

Risk communication

Any exchange of information concerning the existence, nature, form, severity or acceptability of health or environmental risks. Effective risk communication involves determining the types of information that interested and affected parties need and want, and presenting this information to them in a useful and meaningful way.

Decision-Making Framework for Identifying, Assessing and Managing Health Risks. Health Canada, 1 August 2000. (http://www.hc-sc.gc.ca/ahc-asc/pubs/hpfb-dgpsa/risk-risques_cp-pc_e.html, accessed 11 December 2009).

Note: The Erice Declaration on Communicating Drug Safety Information lays out key principles for ethically and effectively communicating information on identi-fied or potential risks. See *Current Challenges in Pharmacovigilance: Report of CIOMS Working Group V.* Geneva, CIOMS, 2001. Appendix 1, pp. 219-220.

Risk estimation

Risk estimation includes the identification of outcomes, the estimation of the magnitude of the associated consequences of these outcomes and the estimation of the probabilities of these outcomes.

Risk analysis, perception and management, The Royal Society, UK, 1992.

Risk evaluation

Risk evaluation is the complex process of determining the significance or value of the identified hazards and estimated risks to those concerned with or affected by the decision. It therefore includes the study of risk perception and the trade-off between perceived risks and perceived benefits. It is defined as the appraisal of the significance of a given quantitative (or where acceptable, qualitative) measure of risk.

Risk analysis, perception and management, The Royal Society, UK, 1992.

Risk management system

A set of pharmacovigilance activities and interventions designed to identify, characterize, prevent or minimize risk relating to medicinal products, and the assess-ment of the effectiveness of those interventions.

Guideline on Risk Management Systems for medicinal products for human use, Vol 9A of Eudralex, Chapter I.3, March 2007. (http://ec.europa.eu/enterprise/pharma-ceuticals/eudralex/vol-9/pdf/vol9_2007-07_upd07.pdf, accessed 11 December 2009).

Serious adverse reaction/Adverse drug reaction

An adverse reaction which results in death, is life-threatening, requires inpatient hospitalization or prolongation of existing hospitalization, results in persistent or significant disability or incapacity, or is a congenital anomaly/birth defect.

Note: Medical events that may not be immediately life-threatening or result in death or hospitalization, but may jeopardize the patient or may require inter-vention to prevent one of the other outcomes listed above, should also usually be considered serious. Examples of such events are: intensive treatment in an emergency room or at home for allergic bronchospasm; blood dyscrasias or convulsions that do not result in hospitalization; or development of drug dependency or drug abuse.

Adapted from *Definitions and Standards for Expedited Reporting, ICH Harmonised Tripartite Guideline, E2A*, Current *Step 4* version, dated 27 October 2004. (http://www.ich.org/LOB/media/MEDIA436.pdf, accessed 11 December 2009)

Signal

Information that arises from one or multiple sources (including observations and experiments), which suggests a new potentially causal association or a new aspect of a known association, between an intervention and an event or set of related events, either adverse or beneficial, that is judged to be of sufficient likelihood to justify verificatory action.

Adapted from: Hauben M, Aronson J.K. Defining "signal" and its subtypes in pharmacovigilance based on a systematic review of previous definitions. *Drug Safety*, 2009, 32:1-12.

Signal detection

The act of looking for and/or identifying signals using event data from any source.

Signal management

A set of activities including signal detection, prioritization and evaluation to determine whether a signal represents a risk which may warrant further assessment, communication or other risk minimization actions in accordance with the medical importance of the issue.

Signal, verified

A signal of suspected causality that has been verified either by its nature or source, e.g. a definitive anecdote or a convincing association that has arisen from a randomized clinical trial or by formal verification studies.

Adapted from: Hauben M, Aronson J.K. Defining "signal" and its subtypes in pharmacovigilance based on a systematic review of previous definitions. *Drug Safety,* 2009, 32:1-12.

Spontaneous report

An unsolicited communication by healthcare professionals or consumers to a company, regulatory authority or other organization that describes one or more suspected adverse drug reactions in a patient who was given one or more medicinal products.

Adapted from *Pharmacovigilance Planning, ICH Harmonised Tripartite Guideline, E2E*, Current *Step 4* version, dated 18 November 2004. (http://www.ich.org/LOB/media/MEDIA1195.pdf, accessed 11 December 2009).

Statistic of disproportionate reporting (SDR)

A numerical result above a preset threshold generated from any data mining algorithm using disproportionality analysis applied to a spontaneous report database. An SDR alerts medical assessors to a specific adverse event reported for a particular medicinal product (drug-event pair) that should be explored further.

Note: SDRs that originate from spontaneous report databases cannot be interpreted as scientific evidence for establishing causality between medicinal products and adverse events, and thus they are distinct from statistical associations that originate from formal epidemiological studies.

Adapted from: *Guideline on the use of statistical signal detection methods in the EudraVigilance data analysis system.* London, Doc. Ref. EMEA/106464/ 2006 rev. 1 (http://www.emea.europa.eu/pdfs/human/phvwp/10646406enfin.pdfm, accessed 11 December 2009).

Targeted medical event (TME)

An adverse event of special interest for a particular medicinal product.

Adapted from: *Guideline on the use of statistical signal detection methods in the EudraVigilance data analysis system.* London, Doc. Ref. EMEA/106464/ 2006 rev. 1 (http://www.emea.europa.eu/pdfs/human/phvwp/10646406enfin.pdfm, accessed 11 December 2009).

Membership and Working Procedures of CIOMS Working Group VIII

CIOMS Working Group VIII on Practical Aspects of Signal Detection in Pharmacovigilance met at a series of six formal meetings in Europe and North America from September 2006 until October 2008. Listed below, followed by a chronology of their work, are 38 senior scientists from drug regulatory authorities, pharmaceutical companies, academia and other institutions who participated in the project.

At the first official meeting held at the European Medicines Agency (EMA) in London in September 2006, the Group agreed on the outline of the project, the working methods and the topics to be addressed. Some new candidate topics were identified during the work and they were included in the report based on discussions within the Working Group.

CIOMS Working Groups I, II, III, IV and V addressed pharmacovigilance issues mostly for the post-authorization phase. CIOMS Working Groups VI and VII focused on the management of safety information from clinical trials and on harmonization of the format and content for periodic safety reporting during clinical trials. It became obvious, however, that signal detection was such an important tool for drug safety monitoring that it required specific consideration and formulation of recommendations on its rational application.

CIOMS Working Group VIII decided to provide points to consider to pharmaceutical companies, regulatory authorities, and international, national or institutional monitoring centres wishing to establish a systematic and holistic strategy to better manage the entire "lifecycle" of a signal. The lifecycle includes signal detection, signal prioritization, and signal evaluation. Moreover, the CIOMS VIII project was designed to focus on the lifecycle of safety signals for pharmaceuticals, including therapeutic biologics. The lifecycle of safety signals in the case of vaccines, however, is covered by the CIOMS/WHO Working Group on Vaccine Pharmacovigilance, which worked in parallel to and interactively with CIOMS WG VIII.

Individual topic chapters and other sections of the CIOMS VIII report were assigned early in the project for consideration and drafting to subgroups with a designated leader. Many participants served on several subgroups. The draft texts and concepts were subsequently reviewed, discussed and debated several times within the entire Working Group, which led to revisions, redrafting and refinements of the text.

After the first meeting at the EMA in London in September 2006, the subsequent meetings were as follows: November 2006 at WHO/CIOMS in Geneva, April 2007 at the Food and Drug Administration in Rockville, Maryland, October 2007 at the Federal Institute for Drugs and Medical Devices (BfArM), Bonn, March 2008 at the French Health Products Safety Agency (Afssaps) in Paris and October 2008 at the Medicines and Healthcare Products Regulatory Agency (MHRA) in London.

Outside experts were invited to critique a draft of the report; they included pharmacovigilance and related specialists from the pharmaceutical industry, academia and health authorities. Their valuable input was incorporated into the final document.

Dr June Raine accepted the role of Chief Editor and compiled and edited the draft consolidated reports and prepared the final manuscript for publication by CIOMS.

Members and advisers of CIOMS Working Group VIII

Name	Organization
June Almenoff	GlaxoSmithKline
Andrew Bate	Uppsala Monitoring Centre (UMC)
Michael Blum*	Wyeth
Anne Castot	French Health Products Safety Agency (Afssaps)
Patrizia Cavazzoni	Eli Lilly
Philippe Close	Novartis
Michael Cook	Wyeth
Gerald Dal Pan	Food and Drug Administration
Gaby Danan	Sanofi Aventis
Paul Dolin	Ingenix
Ralph Edwards*	Uppsala Monitoring Centre (UMC)
Stewart Geary	Eisai
Bill Gregory	Pfizer
Ulrich Hagemann	Federal Institute for Drugs and Medical Devices (BfArM)
Rohan Hammett	Therapeutic Goods Administration (TGA)
Manfred Hauben*	Pfizer
Astrid Herpers	Roche
Christoph Hofman	Bayer Schering AG
William Holden*	Sanofi Pasteur
Sebastian Horn*	Roche
Juhana E. Idänpään-Heikkilä	CIOMS
Chieko Ishiguro*	Pharmaceuticals and Medical Devices Agency (PMDA)
Akira Kawahara	Pharmaceuticals and Medical Devices Agency (PMDA)
Stephen Klincewicz	Johnson & Johnson
Gottfried Kreutz	CIOMS
Lynn Macdonald	Health Canada
François Maignen	EMA
Seiko Masuda*	Pharmaceuticals and Medical Devices Agency (PMDA)
Christiane Michel*	Novartis
Vitali Pool*	Eli Lilly
June Raine	Medicines and Healthcare products Regulatory Agency (MHRA)
Atsuko Shibata	Amgen
Gunilla Sjölin-Forsberg	Medical Products Agency (MPA)
Meredith Y. Smith	Purdue Pharma L.P.
Panos Tsintis*	EMA
Ulrich Vogel	Boehringer-Ingelheim
Jan Venulet	CIOMS
Akiyoshi Uchiyama	Artage

*Adviser

International and national spontaneous reporting system (SRS) databases

Australia – "Blue Card" system

Name of the Regulatory Authority	Therapeutic Goods Administration
Website	http://www.tga.gov.au/problem/index.htm
Name of the database (if applicable)	---
Year of creation of the Pharmacovigilance database	1971
Is the database E2B compliant?	No
Medical terminology used in the database	MedDRA
Drug dictionary used in the database	Proprietary
Total number of ICSRs[1] contained in the database	N/A
Total number of individual cases[2] included in this database	197,298
Number of ICSRs received over the last 3 years	2006: 8614 2005: 9840 2004: 9520
Country of origin of the reports	National spontaneous case reports
Proportion of serious case reports	N/A
Origin of the reports	Health care professionals Patients / consumers Reports from Pharmaceutical Companies Regional health departments
Type of reports captured in the database	Spontaneous reports
Type of products captured in the database	(New) chemical entities Biological medicinal products[3] Vaccines Blood products[4] complementary medicines (e.g. herbal / vitamin / mineral)
Phase of development covered by the database	POST-authorization / POST-marketing
Is the information (or part of this information) made public or available via a FOI (freedom of information) program?	Yes
Quantitative method(s) of signal detection used on the database	PRR
Criteria which are used to define a signal of disproportionate reporting /signal in the database	N/A
Does the database incorporate a formal causality assessment for each report?	Yes. 4 levels, similar to WHO classification: Certain / Probable / Possible / Unclear

Canada – The Health Canada adverse reaction reporting system database for marketed health products (Canada Vigilance)

Name of the Regulatory Authority	Health Canada
Website	http://www.hc-sc.gc.ca/dhp-mps/medeff/ databasdon/index_e.html
Name of the database (if applicable)	Canada Vigilance (upgrade of the previous Canadian Adverse Drug Reaction Information System (CADRIS)).
Year of creation of the Pharmacovigilance database	Contains data going back to 1965.
Is the database E2B compliant?	Yes
Medical terminology used in the database	MedDRA (since January 2008)
Drug dictionary used in the database	Proprietary
Total number of ICSRs contained in the database	N/A
Total number of individual cases included in this database	211,500 domestic cases in the database (December 2007)
Number of ICSRs received over the last 3 years	2007: 17,300 2006: 14,500 2005: 15,000
Country of origin of the reports	National spontaneous case reports
Proportion of serious case reports	Percentage of serious: approx. 66% (in 2006) Percentage of non-serious: approx. 34% (in 2006)
Origin of the reports	Health care professionals Patients / consumers Reports from Pharmaceutical Companies
Type of reports captured in the database	Spontaneous reports Literature Observational studies The majority of the reports are spontaneous reports. There are approximately 5% of reports (from MAH) which resulted from post-marketing (phase IV) studies or reports for comparator drugs from clinical trials
Type of products captured in the database	(New) chemical entities Biological medicinal products Blood products Natural Health Products
Phase of development covered by the database	POST-authorization / POST-marketing
Is the information (or part of this information) made public or available via a FOI (freedom of information) program?	Yes. A subset of the database is posted on the Health Canada website. Data can also be requested under the authority of the Canadian Access to Information (ATI) http://www.hc-sc.gc.ca/dhp-mps/medeff/ databasdon/index_e.html
Quantitative method(s) of signal detection used on the database	The database has the functionality for quantative analysis using EGBM, BCPNN, PRR and ROR
Criteria which are used to define a signal of disproportionate reporting /signal in the database	N/A
Does the database incorporate a formal causality assessment for each report?	No

Canada – The Canadian Adverse Events Following Immunization Surveillance System (CAEFISS) database

Name of the Regulatory Authority	Public Health Agency of Canada
Website	http://www.phac-aspc.gc.ca/im/vs-sv/caefiss_e.html
Name of the database (if applicable)	Canadian Adverse Events Following Immunization Surveillance System
Year of creation of the Pharmacovigilance database	1987
Is the database E2B compliant?	N/A
Medical terminology used in the database	N/A
Drug dictionary used in the database	N/A
Total number of ICSRs contained in the database	N/A
Total number of individual cases included in this database	N/A
Number of ICSRs received over the last 3 years	N/A
Country of origin of the reports	National spontaneous case reports
Proportion of serious case reports	N/A
Origin of the reports	Health care professionals (mainly public health nurses and physicians)
Type of reports captured in the database	N/A
Type of products captured in the database	Vaccines
Phase of development covered by the database	N/A
Is the information (or part of this information) made public or available via a FOI (freedom of information) program?	Data can be requested under the authority of the Canadian Access to Information Act (ATI)
Quantitative method(s) of signal detection used on the database	N/A
Criteria which are used to define a signal of disproportionate reporting /signal in the database	N/A
Does the database incorporate a formal causality assessment for each report?	No but a multidisciplinary group called the Advisory Committee on Causality Assessment (ACCA) has been established to review all case reports meeting criteria for severity or "unexpectedness". Each case is reviewed using the WHO-UMC (World Health Organization-Uppsala Monitoring Centre) causality assessment criteria.

European Union – EudraVigilance

Name of the Regulatory Authority	European Medicines Agency
Website	http://eudravigilance.ema.europa.eu/highres.htm
Name of the database (if applicable)	EudraVigilance (Human)[5]
Year of creation of the Pharmacovigilance database	1 December 2001. EudraVigilance is a data processing network created and maintained by the EMA. EudraVigilance was introduced by Regulation (EEC) No 2309/93, while electronic reporting of adverse reaction reports for marketed products became mandatory in the EU on 20 November 2005.
Is the database E2B compliant?	Yes (transactional database)
Medical terminology used in the database	MedDRA
Drug dictionary used in the database	Proprietary (EVMPD)
Total number of ICSRs contained in the database	More than 1,000,000
Total number of individual cases included in this database	N/A
Number of ICSRs received over the last 3 years	2006: 284,000 2005: 160,000 2004: 94,000
Country of origin of the reports	All serious adverse drug reactions from the EU, serious unexpected from outside the EU
Proportion of serious case reports	all reports are serious
Origin of the reports	Health care professionals Reports from Pharmaceutical Companies
Type of reports captured in the database	Spontaneous reports Literature Compassionate use Registries Observational studies Interventional clinical trials
Type of products captured in the database	(New) chemical entities Biological medicinal products Vaccines Blood products Reports for all medicinal products according to Directive 2001/83/EC (i.e. new therapies, herbal and homeopathic remedies, radiopharmaceuticals, etc ...)
Phase of development covered by the database	POST-authorization / POST-marketing PRE-authorization / PRE-marketing
Is the information (or part of this information) made public or available via a FOI (freedom of information) program?	Not yet. In accordance with the EU legislation, appropriate level of access to EudraVigilance will be given in accordance with the data protection and commercially confidential nature of the information contained in the database.
Quantitative method(s) of signal detection used on the database	PRR
Criteria which are used to define a signal of disproportionate reporting /signal in the database	The lower bound of the 95% confidence interval greater or equal to one and $n \geq 3$ or The PRR > 2, $\chi 2 > 4$ and $n \geq 3$.
Does the database incorporate a formal causality assessment for each report?	No

France – The French Pharmacovigilance System Spontaneous Reports database

Name of the Regulatory Authority	AFSSAPS
Website	http://agmed.sante.gouv.fr/
Name of the database (if applicable)	ANPV
Year of creation of the Pharmacovigilance database	1985 (SOS), upgraded in 1995 and 2007
Is the database E2B compliant?	Yes (since 2005)
Medical terminology used in the database	MedDRA
Drug dictionary used in the database	Proprietary (Codex)
Total number of ICSRs contained in the database	319,027 This figure takes into account only those cases transmitted by the 31 French Regional centres; reports from pharmaceutical companies are not currently entered into the database.
Total number of individual cases included in this database	316,548
Number of ICSRs received over the last 3 years	2006: 20993 2005: 19258 2004: 19947
Country of origin of the reports	National spontaneous case reports
Proportion of serious case reports	Percentage of serious 35% Percentage of non-serious 65% Seriousness taken into account only since 1995. The current proportion is approximately 50-50%.
Origin of the reports	Health care professionals Reports from Pharmaceutical Companies (reports from pharmaceutical companies will be included in the database from the end of 2007 onwards).
Type of reports captured in the database	Spontaneous reports Compassionate use Observational studies
Type of products captured in the database	(New) chemical entities Biological medicinal products Vaccines Blood products
Phase of development covered by the database	POST-authorization / POST-marketing
Is the information (or part of this information) made public or available via a FOI (freedom of information) program?	No
Quantitative method(s) of signal detection used on the database	No signal detection method has been implemented on the database, but will be in the future
Criteria which are used to define a signal of disproportionate reporting /signal in the database	N/A
Does the database incorporate a formal causality assessment for each report?	Yes (French causality assessment method, Begaud *et al.*).

Japan – PMDA / MHLW database

Name of the Regulatory Authority	The Pharmaceuticals and Medical Devices Agency (PMDA) / Ministry of Health, Labour and Welfare (MHLW)
Website	http://www.pmda.go.jp/english/index.html
Name of the database (if applicable)	ADR information management system
Year of creation of the Pharmacovigilance database	27 October 2003
Is the database E2B compliant?	Yes (see table below)
Medical terminology used in the database	J-MedDRA
Drug dictionary used in the database	Proprietary
Total number of ICSRs contained in the database	About 647,000 (164,000 domestic reports)
Total number of individual cases included in this database	About 412,000 (83,000 domestic report)
Number of ICSRs received over the last 3 years (Japanese Fiscal year)	2006: about 210,000 2005: about 193,000 2004: about 171,000
Country of origin of the reports	National spontaneous case reports (Health care professionals and pharmaceutical companies) Foreign case reports (from pharmaceutical companies)
Proportion of serious case reports	Pre-marketing: only serious ADR. Post-marketing: The data from 2003 to 2004 contain also moderate case reports. But after 2005, only serious cases are reported under the revision to the law.
Origin of the case reports (see table below)	Health care professionals Reports from Pharmaceutical Companies
Type of case reports captured in the database (see table below)	Spontaneous reports Literature Compassionate use Registries Observational studies Interventional clinical trials
Type of products captured in the database	(New) chemical entities (incl. OTC medicines) Biological medicinal products Vaccines Blood products Herbals
Phase of development covered by the database	POST-authorization / POST-marketing PRE-authorization / PRE-marketing
Is the information (or part of this information) made public or available via a FOI (freedom of information) program?	Yes (part of this information). A subset is published on the PMDA website http://www.info.pmda.go.jp/ (in Japanese)
Quantitative method(s) of signal detection used on the database	PRR, BCPNN, MGPS, ROR, SPRT, GPS have been used on a trial basis. Final stage of development of these methods in order to start running them in 2009.
Criteria which are used to define a signal of disproportionate reporting /signal in the database	Under consideration
Does the database incorporate a formal causality assessment for each report?	Yes (Proprietary classification). There is a causality assessment for each report mainly for those unlisted serious ADR. In the near future, it is planned to conduct causality assessments for each report about broader ADR in post marketing.

Table 1: case reports reported to the ADR information management system

Reporter	post/pre marketing	report contents	format
Pharmaceutical company	post/pre	domestic infection	ICSR(E2B)
	post/pre	domestic ADR	ICSR(E2B)
	post/pre	foreign infection	ICSR(E2B)
	post/pre	foreign ADR	ICSR(E2B)
	post/pre	research paper on infection	
	post/pre	research paper on ADR	
	post/pre	measures taken in foreign country	
	post/pre	quasi drug and cosmetics	
Medical professional	Post	domestic infection and ADR	ICSR

The Netherlands – Lareb database

Name of the Regulatory Authority	Netherlands Pharmacovigilance Centre Lareb (on behalf of the Dutch MEB)
Website	http://www.lareb.nl/
Name of the database (if applicable)	Lareb2002
Year of creation of the Pharmacovigilance database	Data since 1985, Current database operational since 2002
Is the database E2B compliant?	Yes
Medical terminology used in the database	MedDRA
Drug dictionary used in the database	G-standaard (Drug dictionary from the Dutch Pharmacist Association)
Total number of ICSRs contained in the database	Appr 60,000 (follow up information included in the original report)
Total number of individual cases included in this database	
Number of ICSRs received over the last 3 years	2006: appr 6300 2005: appr 6300 2004: appr 5000
Country of origin of the reports	National spontaneous case reports
Proportion of serious case reports	N/A
Origin of the reports	Health care professionals Patients / consumers Reports from Pharmaceutical Companies
Type of reports captured in the database	Spontaneous reports Literature (via MAH)
Type of products captured in the database	(New) chemical entities Biological medicinal products Vaccines Herbals, homeopathy
Phase of development covered by the database	POST-authorization / POST-marketing
Is the information (or part of this information) made public or available via a FOI (freedom of information) program?	Yes
Quantitative method(s) of signal detection used on the database	Reporting Odds Ratio
Criteria which are used to define a signal of disproportionate reporting /signal in the database	Lower limit 95% CI >1 and more than 3 reports, but clinical information is decisive
Does the database incorporate a formal causality assessment for each report?	Yes (Naranjo algorithm)

Sweden – SWEDIS database (SWE-WEB) Medicinal Products Agency

Name of the Regulatory Authority	Medical Products Agency
Website	http://sweweb.mpa.se
Name of the database (if applicable)	SWEDIS
Year of creation of the Pharmacovigilance database	Data since 1965, Current database operational since 1974
Is the database E2B compliant?	Yes
Medical terminology used in the database	WHO-ART. Reports transferred to the EudraVigilance database are mapped to be E2B compliant.
Drug dictionary used in the database	SWEDIS
Total number of ICSRs contained in the database	Approx 105,000 (by year 2007). Follow up information included in the original report
Total number of individual cases included in this database	Approx 105,000 (2007)
Number of ICSRs received over the last 3 years	2007: 4,817 2006: 5,130 2005: 4,071 2004: 4,124
Country of origin of the reports	National spontaneous case reports
Proportion of serious case reports	32 per cent
Origin of the reports	Mainly health care professionals
Type of reports captured in the database	Spontaneous reports
Type of products captured in the database	(New) chemical entities Biological medicinal products Vaccines Herbals, homeopathy
Phase of development covered by the database	POST-authorization / POST-marketing
Is the information (or part of this information) made public or available via a FOI (freedom of information) program?	Yes, on request
Quantitative method(s) of signal detection used on the database	Mainly Proportional Reporting Ratio in routine work. BCPNN has been used on a research basis.
Criteria which are used to define a signal of disproportionate reporting /signal in the database	Lower limit 95% CI >1 and usually more than 3 reports, but clinical information is decisive
Does the database incorporate a formal causality assessment for each report?	Yes. 5 levels, similar to WHO classification: Certain / Probable / Possible / Unlikely/ Unclassifiable

The United Kingdom – "Yellow Card" database (Sentinel)

Name of the Regulatory Authority	Medicines and Healthcare products Regulatory Agency
Website	http://www.mhra.gov.uk/index.htm and http://yellowcard.mhra.gov.uk/
Name of the database (if applicable)	Sentinel
Year of creation of the Pharmacovigilance database	Sentinel was deployed in 2006. Previous records dating back to 1963 were held on the ADROIT database (1991-2006)
Is the database E2B compliant?	Yes
Medical terminology used in the database	MedDRA
Drug dictionary used in the database	Proprietary
Total number of ICSRs contained in the database	571894 UK Spontaneous Cases
Total number of individual cases included in this database	N/A
Number of ICSRs received over the last 3 years	2006: 21899 UK spontaneous cases 2005: 21979 UK spontaneous cases 2004: 19988 UK spontaneous cases
Country of origin of the reports	National spontaneous case reports Foreign case reports (EU and non-EU)
Proportion of serious case reports	Percentage of serious 70-80% Percentage of non-serious 20-30%
Origin of the reports	Health care professionals Patients / consumers Reports from Pharmaceutical Companies Non-commercial Clinical Trials
Type of reports captured in the database	Spontaneous reports Literature Compassionate use Registries Observational studies Interventional clinical trials
Type of products captured in the database	(New) chemical entities Biological medicinal products Vaccines Herbals/ Unlicensed Products
Phase of development covered by the database	POST-authorization / POST-marketing PRE-authorization / PRE-marketing
Is the information (or part of this information) made public or available via a FOI (freedom of information) program?	Yes
Quantitative method(s) of signal detection used on the database	MGPS
Criteria which are used to define a signal of disproportionate reporting /signal in the database	A combination of a signal selection threshold for the empirical Bayes MGPS (at least 3 reports of the drug-ADR combination with 1 report received in the previous week, EBGM $\geq$ 2.5 and EB05 $\geq$ 1.8) and additional fatal, paediatric and parent-child and drug interaction reports is used to identify possible signals. A list of 'alert' terms has also been created comprising of serious reactions of concern such as toxic epidermal necrolysis which identifies further additional reports for evaluation.
Does the database incorporate a formal causality assessment for each report?	No

The United States – Adverse Event Reporting System (AERS) database

Name of the Regulatory Authority	U.S. Food and Drug Administration
Website	http://www.fda.gov/medwatch/ and http:// www.fda.gov/cder/aers/default.htm
Name of the database (if applicable)	AERS (Adverse Event Reporting System)
Year of creation of the Pharmacovigilance database	1969 (re-engineered in 1997)
Is the database E2B compliant?	Yes
Medical terminology used in the database	MedDRA
Drug dictionary used in the database	CDER, FDA
Total number of ICSRs contained in the database	Approximately 4 millions
Total number of individual cases included in this database	Approximately 3.4 millions
Number of ICSRs received over the last 3 years	2006: approx. 350,000 2005: approx. 330,000 2004: approx. 310,000
Country of origin of the reports	U.S. and worldwide foreign countries. Only serious and unlabelled adverse event reports from foreign sources are required for the sponsor to submit to FDA.
Proportion of serious case reports	Percentage of serious outcome reports is 60% (approximately for all years combined) Percentage of non-serious outcome reports is 40% (approximately for all years combined)
Origin of the reports	Health care professionals Patients / consumers Reports from Pharmaceutical Companies Regulatory authority reports received by pharmaceutical companies are submitted to FDA by pharmaceutical companies.
Type of reports captured in the database	Spontaneous reports Literature Compassionate use (reported as study report) Registries (reported as study report) Observational studies (reported as study report) Interventional clinical trials (reported as study report) Only serious, unexpected adverse experience reports from literature are required for the pharmaceutical companies to submit to FDA. Only serious, unexpected adverse experiences from studies if there is a reasonable possibility that the drug or biologic product caused the adverse experiences are required for the pharmaceutical companies to submit to FDA.

Name of the Regulatory Authority	U.S. Food and Drug Administration
Type of products captured in the database	(New) chemical entities Biological medicinal products Blood products All products approved for marketing in the U.S. are captured in the database. Over-the-Counter (OTC) products marketed under the Monograph without approved applications are captured as well.
Phase of development covered by the database	POST-authorization / POST-marketing
Is the information (or part of this information) made public or available via a FOI (freedom of information) program?	Yes. Names of patients, healthcare professionals, hospitals and geographical identifiers in adverse drug experience reports are not releasable to the public under FDA's public information or FOI regulations.
Quantitative method(s) of signal detection used on the database	MGPS Safety signal detections from AERS usually are generated by manual review of case reports of interest. Disproportionate observation or analysis of AERS data based on routine monitoring or report frequency counts of products may be used occasionally. Recently, data mining or disproportionate analysis scores of AERS data using MGPS methodology is utilized routinely to enhance the monitoring and signal detection process. Clinical review of case reports is always followed to evaluate the potential signals identified from data mining.
Criteria which are used to define a signal of disproportionate reporting /signal in the database	Based on the methodology, theoretically any data mining scores (EB05) greater than 1.0 is potentially a signal for further investigation. CDER/FDA has routinely used EB05 scores greater than 2.0 more often to initiate any significant investigation. http://www.fda.gov/cder/aers/extract.htm
Does the database incorporate a formal causality assessment for each report?	No

The United States – The Vaccine Adverse Events Reporting System (VAERS) database

Name of the Regulatory Authority	U.S. Food and Drug Administration
Website	http://vaers.hhs.gov/
Name of the database (if applicable)	VAERS (Adverse Event Reporting System)
Year of creation of the Pharmacovigilance database	1990
Is the database E2B compliant?	Not yet
Medical terminology used in the database	MedDRA
Drug dictionary used in the database	Proprietary
Total number of ICSRs contained in the database	212,878
Total number of individual cases included in this database	206,536
Number of ICSRs received over the last 3 years	2006: approx. 19 473 2005: approx. 17 761 2004: approx. 16 710
Country of origin of the reports	National spontaneous case reports Foreign case reports (Usually serious unlabelled from manufacturers).
Proportion of serious case reports	Percentage of serious outcome reports is 14.5% Percentage of non-serious outcome reports is 85.5%
Origin of the reports	Health care professionals Patients / consumers Reports from Pharmaceutical Companies
Type of reports captured in the database	Spontaneous reports Literature from manufacturers Interventional clinical trials (reported as study report) Post-marketing studies reports for serious unlabelled AEs if the re is a reasonable possibility that the product caused the AE.
Type of products captured in the database	Vaccines
Phase of development covered by the database	POST-authorization / POST-marketing
Is the information (or part of this information) made public or available via a FOI (freedom of information) program?	Yes http://vaers.hhs.gov/scripts/data.cfm
Quantitative method(s) of signal detection used on the database	PRR MGPS
Criteria which are used to define a signal of disproportionate reporting /signal in the database	PRR > 2 with n> 3 and chi-square > 4 EB05 > 2
Does the database incorporate a formal causality assessment for each report?	No

WHO (Uppsala Monitoring Centre) – Vigibase

Name of the Regulatory Authority	The Uppsala Monitoring Centre
Website	http://www.who-umc.org/
Name of the database (if applicable)	Vigibase (WHO International database)
Year of creation of the Pharmacovigilance database	1968
Is the database E2B compliant?	Yes
Medical terminology used in the database	WHO-ART and MedDRA
Drug dictionary used in the database	WHO Drug Dictionary
Total number of ICSRs contained in the database	N/A
Total number of individual cases included in this database	Approx. 4,000,000
(Number of ICSRs received over the last 3 years) Number of ICSRs processed over the last 3 years	2006: 385,924 2005: 451,189 2004: 301,931
	Spontaneous case reports from WHO Drug Monitoring Program member countries
Proportion of serious case reports	Percentage of serious 9.4% Percentage of non-serious 89.3% (Percentage not specified 1.3%)
Origin of the reports	Health care professionals Patients / consumers Reports from Pharmaceutical Companies (Vigibase accept ADR-reports from the National Centres which can receive reports from all categories mentioned above).
Type of reports captured in the database	Mostly spontaneous reports
Type of products captured in the database	(New) chemical entities Biological medicinal products Vaccines Blood products Herbal and Homeopathic remedies
Phase of development covered by the database	POST-authorization / POST-marketing
Is the information (or part of this information) made public or available via a FOI (freedom of information) program?	No
Quantitative method(s) of signal detection used on the database	BCPNN
Criteria which are used to define a signal of disproportionate reporting /signal in the database	IC025 newly greater than zero as well as triage filters as defined in Stahl M, Lindquist M, Edwards IR, and Brown EG. Introducing triage logic as a new strategy for the detection of signals in the WHO Drug Monitoring Database. Pharmacoepidemiol Drug Saf 2004; 13: 355-63.
Does the database incorporate a formal causality assessment for each report?	Yes (WHO causality)

[1] The number of ICSRs includes all the reports received by the organization, both initial and follow-up reports.
[2] An individual case is a single occurrence containing the original and all the follow-up reports.
[3] Excluding vaccines
[4] This refers to the blood derived medicinal products excluding labile blood products
[5] EudraVigilance also contains a module for veterinary medicinal products.

Table 2. Database Resources Stratified by Country. Listing modified from an informal list prepared by members of the International Society for Pharmacoepidemiology (ISPE), originally dated 27 January 2005.

British Columbia Healthcare Utilization Databases	Canada	http://www.gov.bc.ca/healthservices
Population Health Research Unit	Canada	http://phru.medicine.dal.ca
Saskatchewan Health Databases	Canada	http://www.health.gov.sk.ca/
Odense University Pharmacoepidemiological Database (OPED)	Denmark	http://www.sdu.dk/health/research/units/clinpharm.php
Pharmacoepidemiological Prescription Databases of North Jutland (PDNJ)	Denmark	http://www.clin-epi.dk
Finland Medical Record Linkage System	Finland	
PEDIANET	Italy	http://www.pedianet.it
Sistema Informativo Sanitario Regionale Database-FVG region (FVG)	Italy	
Health Insurance Review Agency Database (HIRA)	Korea	http://www.hira.or.kr
Integrated Primary Care Information Database	Netherlands	http://www.ipci.nl
InterAction Database (IADB)	Netherlands	
PHARMO Record Linkage System	Netherlands	http://www.pharmo.nl
Medicines Monitoring Unit (MEMO)	Scotland	http://www.dundee.ac.uk/memo
Primary Care Clinical Informatics Unit-Research (PCCIU-R)	Scotland	http://www.abdn.ac.uk/general_practice/research/special/pcciu.shtml
Base de datos para la Investigacion Farmacoepidemiologica en Atencion Primaria (BIFAP)	Spain	ttp://www.bifap.org/
Swedish Centre for Epidemiology	Sweden	http://www.sos.se/epc/epceng.htm#epid
General Practice Research Database (GPRD)	UK	http://www.gprd.com/
IMS Disease Analyzer (MediPlus)	UK	http://research.imshealth.com
Prescription Event Monitoring (PEM) Database	UK	http://www.dsru.org/main.html
The Health Improvement Network (THIN)	UK	http://www.epic-uk.org
BRIDGE Database of Databases	US/Europe	http://www.dgiinc.org/html/frameset.htm
Boston Collaborative Drug Surveillance Program (BCDSP)-GPRD	US	http://www.bcdsp.org
Case-Control Surveillance Study	US	http://www.bu.edu/slone/
Constella Health Sciences	US	http://www.constellagroup.com/health_sciences/
Framingham Heart Study Database	US	http://www.nhlbi.nih.gov/about/framingham/index.html
Group Health Cooperative of Puget Sound	US	http://www.centerforhealthstudies.org/
Harvard Pilgrim Health Care	US	http://www.harvardpilgrim.org

Name	Country	URL
Healthcare Cost & Utilization Project (HCUP)	US	http://www.ahrq.gov/data/hcup/
Healthcore (Wellpoint/Blue Cross/Blue Shield)	US	http://www.healthcore.com
Henry Ford Health System (HFHS)	US	http://www.henryfordhealth.org
HMO Research Network (HMORN)	US	http://www.hmoresearchnetwork.org
IMS LifeLink	US	http://secure.imshealth.com/public/structure/ dispcontent/1,2779,1203-1203-143177,00.html
IMS National Disease and Therapeutic Index	US	http://www.imshealth.com/ims/portal/front/ articleC/0,2777,6599_44000160_44022368,00.html
Ingenix Epidemiology – UnitedHealthcare	US	http://www.epidemiology.com
Integrated Healthcare Information Solutions (IHCIS)	US	http://www.ihcis.com
Kaiser Permanente Medical Care Programs	US	http://www.dor.kaiser.org/
Kaiser Permanente Northwest	US	http://www.kpchr.org/public/studies/studies.aspx
Lovelace Health and Environmental Epi Program	US	http://www.lrri.org/cr/cpor.html
MarketScan	US	http://www.medstat.com/1products/marketscan.asp
Medicaid Databases	US	
Medical Expenditure Panel Survey (MEPS)	US	http://www.ahrq.gov/data/mepsix.htm
National Ambulatory Medical Care Survey	US	http://www.cdc.gov/nchs
National Death Index	US	http://www.cdc.gov/nchs/r&d/ndi/ndi.htm
National Health and Nutrition Examination Survey	US	http://www.cdc.gov/nchs/nhanes.htm
National Health Care Survey	US	http://www.cdc.gov/nchs/nhcs.htm
National Health Interview Study	US	http://www.cdc.gov/nchs/nhis.htm
National Hospital Discharge Survey	US	http://www.cdc.gov/nchs/about/major/hdasd/nhds.htm
National Natality Survey	US	http://www.cdc.gov/nchs
National Nursing Home Survey	US	http://www.cdc.gov/nchs/about/major/nnhsd/nnhsd.htm
NDC Health's Intelligent Health Repository	US	http://www.ndchealth.com/index.asp
Nurses Health Study	US	http://www.channing.harvard.edu/nhs/
PharMetrics	US	http://www.pharmetrics.com
Pregnancy Health Interview Study	US	http://www.bu.edu/slone/
Slone Survey	US	http://www.bu.edu/slone/
Solucient	US	http://www.solucient.com/
Surveillance Epidemiology & End Results (SEER)	US	http://seer.cancer.gov/
Vaccine Safety Datalink	US	http://www.cdc.gov/nip/vacsafe/
Veterans Administration Databases	US	http://www.virec.research.med.va.gov

Appendix 4

Table A: Epidemiologic studies

STUDY TYPE	LEVEL OF INFERENCE	STUDY TYPE EXAMPLE	POSSIBLE INFERENCE
OBSERVATIONAL	Non-inferential (descriptive)	Case reports	Suggestion of an association
	Population	Surveillance (incidence, mortality)	Documentation of baseline disease burden, exploratory hypotheses
		Ecologic (correlation study)	Coarse verification of correlation between exposure and disease
	Individual	Cross-sectional	Correlation between exposure (or marker) and disease without regard to latency
		Case-control	Correlation between exposure (or marker) and disease with improved understanding of latency; rare disease
		Cohort	Correlation between exposure (or marker) and disease with improved understanding of latency; rare exposures
EXPERIMENTAL	Individual	In general, randomized controlled trial	'Unbiased' assessment of the relation between exposure and disease/occurrence of a reaction

Table B: Variations of main epidemiologic study design

STUDY DESIGN	MAIN FEATURE
Cohort study	Subjects recruited on the basis of exposure to drug or vaccine; comparative incidence rates of AEs
Case-control study	Subjects recruited on the basis of the presence of disease or other outcome; OR of association is calculated
Nested case-control study	Cases and controls are selected from a pre-existing cohort; more efficient estimator of RR
Case cohort study	Case-control variation in which controls are not matched to cases but selected randomly at beginning of follow-up (and they may become cases)
Case crossover study	Case-control variation used when a brief exposure causes a transient increase in acute, rare outcome
Case-time-control study	Case crossover modification which tries to separate time effect from drug effect
Case coverage study	Essentially an unmatched case-control design with the entire population (including cases) as controls
Self-controlled case series	Uses cases as their own controls at different time periods; rates during exposed periods compared to rates during unexposed periods
Registry	Routine disease or drug/vaccine specific data collected continuously or repeatedly that can be related back to a specified population base
Meta-analysis	Statistical combination of results from several studies that individually lack enough power to demonstrate a small but important effect
Prescription event monitoring	Non-interventional, observational cohort form of post-marketing surveillance of drugs in the UK
Drug utilization study	The study of prescribing, dispensing, administering, marketing, and ingesting of drugs in society, with emphasis on the resulting medical, social, and economic consequences
Large simple safety study	Randomized clinical trial approach using much simplified protocol, data collection and analytic techniques; mimics clinical practice; further assessment of benefits and risks

Appendix 5

Points to consider regarding differences between vaccines and drugs in signal detection

With signal detection, there is a substantial overlap of vaccines and drugs in the methods and approaches used. Nonetheless, vaccines present some important differences worthy of special attention. This brief appendix presents points to consider for those undertaking signal detection for prophylactic vaccines.

The development of vaccines and their settings of post-licensure use lead to several special issues. In general, vaccine pre-licensure trials are substantially larger than those for drugs and consequently are powered to detect rarer adverse events.

Universal immunization and public communication of safety signals

The goal of ensuring the safety of vaccines leads to the institution of rigorous signal detection efforts. Vaccines are often required by authorities for school attendance or other reasons, resulting in greater than 90% coverage rates; this is sometimes called "universal immunization". Universal immunization programs have successfully controlled or eliminated multiple infectious diseases. However, certain publicized adverse events following immunization (AEFI) based on weak scientific data have led to concerns followed by substantial decreases in vaccination coverage rates and subsequent increases in incidence of vaccine preventable disease (1). The lack of an alternative vaccine can exacerbate such situations. Consequently, public communication of unconfirmed vaccine safety signals should take into account the potential effects on vaccination coverage as well as the benefits (e.g. adverse event case ascertainment) and any other risks of communicating the signal.

Implications of standard ages at vaccination

Paediatric vaccines are often recommended to be administered at specific ages, predominantly to healthy infants and children. Multiple diseases and conditions have characteristic ages at onset that may occur contemporaneously, or nearly so, with recommended vaccinations. Even in the absence of a causal association of a vaccination with a disease, a temporal association may be observed. For example, if a disease's median age of onset and diagnosis occurred at age 15 months, and if the disease were not causally associated with a vaccination recommended at age 15 months, one would nonetheless at a minimum expect spontaneous reports of that disease being associated with vaccination. Some investigators or members of the public might then posit a causal association even though none exists. On the other hand, contemporaneous occurrence of the recommended age of vaccination and the natural onset of disease does not by itself rule out a causal association or a triggering effect, and further investigation may be warranted depending on the totality of the available information.

Settings of vaccine administration

Vaccine administration settings may differ from those for drugs. Examples of such, where physicians are often absent, include public settings such as vaccination clinics, pharmacies and schools. Consequently, the nature of adverse event reports following vaccination in these settings may differ in both quantity and quality from the settings where drugs traditionally are administered or prescribed. For example, in mass vaccination programs there may be clusters of vasovagal-like episodes, some involving syncope that may be mistakenly reported as other, more severe conditions without medical confirmation (2). In contrast, a new serious adverse event may first come to attention during a mass vaccination campaign as occurred in 1976 with Guillain-Barré syndrome following swine flu vaccine in the USA (3).

Live attenuated viral or bacterial vaccines

In clear contrast to drugs, some vaccines are composed of attenuated viruses or bacteria that are intended to cause mild infections that induce protective immunity. Rarely, these vaccine-induced infections result in serious disease. Investigation of such infections is important. Identification of the pathogenic organism and determining whether it is vaccine strain or "wild type" through culture, DNA-based techniques or other methods can be crucial to linking the vaccine to the adverse event.

Vaccine components included for antigenic or non-antigenic attributes

Antigens in vaccines are intended to elicit a protective immune response in the vaccinee. However, there exists the possibility that vaccination may inadvertently elicit an unintended and pathologic immune or autoimmune response (e.g. immune thrombocytopenic purpura following measles-mumps-rubella vaccination). In addition, components of vaccines that are included for attributes other than their antigenic value – such as adjuvants intended to augment the immune response to vaccine antigens, sterilizing agents and stabilizers – may lead to adverse events distinct from those typically associated with drugs. These components may be present in different vaccines protecting against widely varying diseases, and this potential should be taken into account in data analyses.

Combination vaccines and simultaneous administration of multiple vaccines

Vaccines are not only formulated in fixed combinations (e.g. diphtheria-tetanus-pertussis (DTP) vaccine) but also multiple vaccines are frequently administered simultaneously at different body sites. Consequently, in situations where one vaccine is associated with an adverse event, it may be difficult to determine which of multiple simultaneously administered vaccines underlies the association. Depending on the analytic approach, a co-administered vaccine may be spuriously associated with an adverse event (for example, using automated signal detection approaches, DTP vaccine may be found to be associated with polio, although the disease was due to co-administered oral polio vaccine).

Data analytic issues

Regulatory authorities and vaccine manufacturers maintain spontaneous adverse event report databases which vary in size, diversity of products, case characteristics and countries covered. Spontaneous adverse event report databases may include vaccines only (such as the United States Vaccine Adverse Event Reporting System (VAERS)) or both vaccines and drugs (such as the EU's EudraVigilance). Depending on the type of signal detection task and approach used, and the scientific question being asked, one of these two types of databases may perform better than the other. In a vaccines-only database, particularly in manufacturers' databases, one vaccine may compose a relatively large proportion of the adverse event reports and might skew the analyses. In a mixed drugs-vaccines database, drug reports will usually greatly outnumber vaccine reports, and analyses should take this into account where appropriate. Some of the common differences between groups receiving vaccines and drugs are mentioned in this annex. In the United States databases there are also substantial differences in the proportion of vaccine and drug reports that are categorized as 'serious', about 15% for vaccines and substantially more for drugs (the percentage for drugs may decrease with the widespread implementation of electronic submission). Combining such disparate databases for analysis clearly may be problematic and should be done carefully, taking into account the potential for bias and confounding. Another aspect that differs between vaccines and drugs that may affect signal detection and analyses is the substantially greater number of drugs than vaccines. In addition, in the United States, a much greater proportion of adverse event reports from manufacturers is found in the Adverse Event Reporting System (AERS) than in VAERS. This may result in greater differences in signal detection between company databases and VAERS than between company databases and AERS; analogous situations may exist in other countries or settings. In addition, depending on a report's source, its quality and the potential for obtaining additional follow-up information for assessment of signals may vary.

Additional analytic issues for consideration include: in the setting of universal immunization, signal detection and assessment modalities that utilize unvaccinated persons as a comparison group should take into account the possibility that unvaccinated persons, who may be a small minority, differ systematically from vaccinated persons in ways that may be associated with the adverse event of interest. This potential for confounding should be explicitly addressed. In addition, confounding by indication is a greater concern in drug signal detection than for vaccines because, in general, vaccine recipients are healthier than those who receive drugs. Moreover, vaccines are often used in paediatric populations, whereas drugs are usually used in older people. These differences may affect the choice of appropriate comparison groups and analytic approaches.

In any vaccine adverse event analysis, confounders or sources of bias to be considered include (but are not limited to) age, gender, race/ethnicity, season (e.g. for influenza vaccines), calendar time and country/region; in addition, it is usually desirable to take event seriousness into account.

Possible analyses by class, brand or lot

Whether to analyze vaccines of the same type together and/or separately is an important decision. For example, in a given annual influenza season, an association between Guillain-Barré and the influenza vaccine may be signaled by analyses of all inactivated influenza vaccines combined and/or of each brand of vaccine independently. In addition, analysis by vaccine lot is possible and may be indicated for routine surveillance or in the event of a potential cluster or other lot safety concern.

Small number of doses per vaccine per person

Specific vaccines are usually administered to an individual in a series of a small number of doses (rarely more than four times annually and most often fewer). In contrast, many drugs are administered at least daily, often for extended duration. Vaccines' infrequent dosing schedule and induction of long-term immunity make the use of dechallenge, useful for drug safety assessment, generally not applicable for vaccines; similarly, opportunities for rechallenge are much less frequent for vaccines than for drugs. Safety analyses involving vaccines may need to take into account these differences. Self-control methodologies, in which an individual who has received a product has "exposed" and "unexposed" time windows whose adverse event incidence rates are compared, have particular advantages in hypothesis testing, signal evaluation and possibly in detection as well (4, 5). For drugs administered frequently, "unexposed" time windows after drug initiation appropriate for analysis may be less available.

Automated signal detection

Automated signal detection (sometimes called "data mining") is increasingly used and has some specific considerations in addition to the ones noted above (6, 7). In databases that include both drug and vaccine adverse event reports, investigators should give careful consideration to the choice of the comparison group. For example, a comparison group including drugs may result in the detection of vaccine adverse event signals that relate to vaccines as a class (e.g. fever) and may also identify false signals (e.g. sudden infant death syndrome) or already known mild and expected reactions linked to vaccination (e.g. local injection site reactions). However, simply restricting analyses to vaccines does not solve all problems, and issues highlighted in the Data Analytic Issues and other sections above – such as addressing potential confounding by age, simultaneous administration of multiple vaccines, and other factors – should be taken into account. It may be appropriate to undertake automated signal detection using some analyses of vaccines alone and other analyses including drugs also.

References

1. McIntyre P, Leask J. Improving uptake of MMR vaccine. *British Medical Journal*. 5 April 2008, 336(7647):729-30.

2. Clements CJ. Mass psychogenic illness after vaccination. *Drug Safety*, 2003, 26(9):599-604.

3. Langmuir AD et al. An epidemiologic and clinical evaluation of Guillain-Barré syndrome reported in association with the administration of swine influenza vaccines. *American Journal of Epidemiology*, 1984, 119:841-79.

4. Farrington CP. Control without separate controls: evaluation of vaccine safety using case-only methods. *Vaccine*. 7 May 2004, 22(15-16):2064-70.

5. Davis RL et al. Active surveillance of vaccine safety: a system to detect early signs of adverse events. *Epidemiology*. May 2005, 16(3):336-41.

6. Iskander J et al. The VAERS Team. Data mining in the US using the Vaccine Adverse Event Reporting System. *Drug Safety*, 2006, 29(5):375-84.

7. Banks D et al. Comparing data mining methods on the VAERS database. *Pharmacoepidemiology and Drug Safety*, September 2005, 14(9):601-9.